The Third Population

The Third Population

Aurélien Ducoudray and Jeff Pourquié

The Pennsylvania State University Press
University Park, Pennsylvania

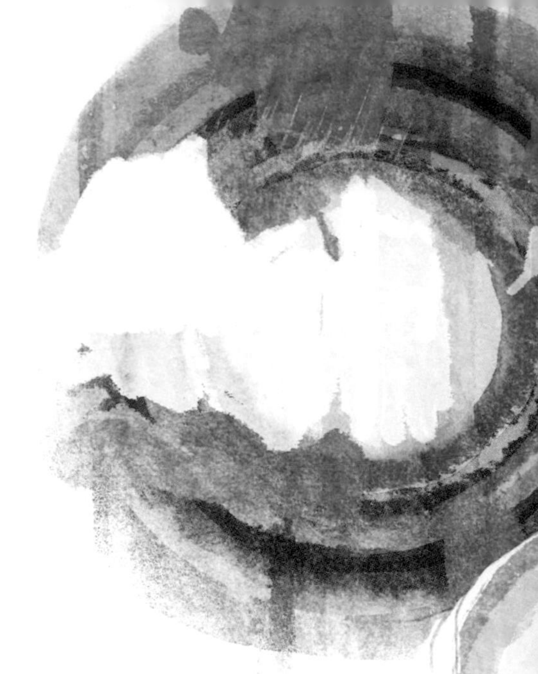

Mental illness is an issue that affects us all.

One in four people is likely to develop a mental illness over the course of his or her life. In 2008, as many as 1.3 million people received treatment in the French psychiatric care system. One percent of our population has schizophrenia; two percent has a mood disorder. Many of our families, neighbors, and friends are affected by mental illness. But for some reason it still frightens us.

Our politicians rarely address mental illness, and when they do, it usually only reinforces the stigma.

That's why this graphic novel is so timely. What better way to combat prejudice than to share in the lives of the mentally ill, even if just for a short time? That's why I have always supported the regionalization of our mental health services and the Marisol Touraine Health Act of 2017. Local mental health councils have also been doing a lot to destigmatize mental illness as they work to provide patients with access to community health services.

This graphic novel highlights an aspect of French psychiatry that has become known the world over. *La psychothérapie institutionnelle*, or institutional psychotherapy, first flourished in the Loir-et-Cher—in Borde with Dr. Oury, in Chesnaie with Dr. Jeangirard, and in the clinic at Saumery. With an approach that some might consider impractical, institutional psychotherapy promotes a lifestyle in which caregivers, patients, and the institution itself can work together to build meaningful human relationships, in spite of the difficulties that mental illness can pose. Even though psychiatric treatment has taken a fair amount of criticism for protocols that have advised the use of drugs, isolation, and restraint, psychoanalysis has also had a deep and abiding respect for its patients, and that's what makes it so therapeutically effective.

This graphic novel embodies that spirit: it reveals the humanity in us all.

Denys Robiliard
Former National Assembly representative specializing in mental health and the future of psychiatry in France

Psychiatric institutions have recently had to face the fact that, in the minds of many, they are seen as places of isolation and seclusion.

In the years following the Second World War, progressive psychiatrists threw open the doors of outmoded asylums for the mentally ill and made some changes. They banned the term "asylum" and proposed a more neutral term, like "psychotherapy center." More recently, and somewhat paradoxically, the process of de-institutionalizing mental health care has disturbed the delicate balance between the inside and the outside worlds of mental illness. The postwar generation of psychiatrists had worked to foster the reciprocal flow of patients out into the community and community members into clinic spaces. But in a classic case of "throwing the baby out with the bath water," the recent reduction of institutional space has meant that patients were discharged and services were either abandoned or, in the best-case scenario, outsourced to external organizations, thus putting psychiatric facilities out of business.

For the past sixty years, Chesnaie has bucked this trend without setting up walls or closing its doors. Always open to the outside world, the clinic's boundaries have been permeable, permitting patient access, for example, to public concerts and seminars, and welcoming within the clinic's walls artists-in-residence or visiting writers and artists. But the institution has also succeeded in maintaining an invisible boundary with the surrounding community, setting aside for those within the clinic the time and space necessary for private moments and social events.

If mental illness plays out as part of a process, it is also a sort of trauma. Nervous responses to the strange, abnormal, and incomprehensible can have a profound effect on those who are ill. When others respond to psychiatric patients with fear or sadness, even if unintentionally, it can cause additional suffering. Moreover, the very fact of being in treatment, even when the care is excellent, can affect a patient's self-esteem. Nevertheless, having some agency over one's treatment is important and constructive work that requires access to a wide range of psychotherapeutic tools, from group therapy to seemingly unrelated tasks, such as helping to make a meal for the community.

With humor and sensitivity, this book offers useful insight into the workings of a clinic where institutional psychotherapy is put into practice.

Dr. Jean-Louis Place
Medical Director
The Chesnaie Psychiatric Clinic

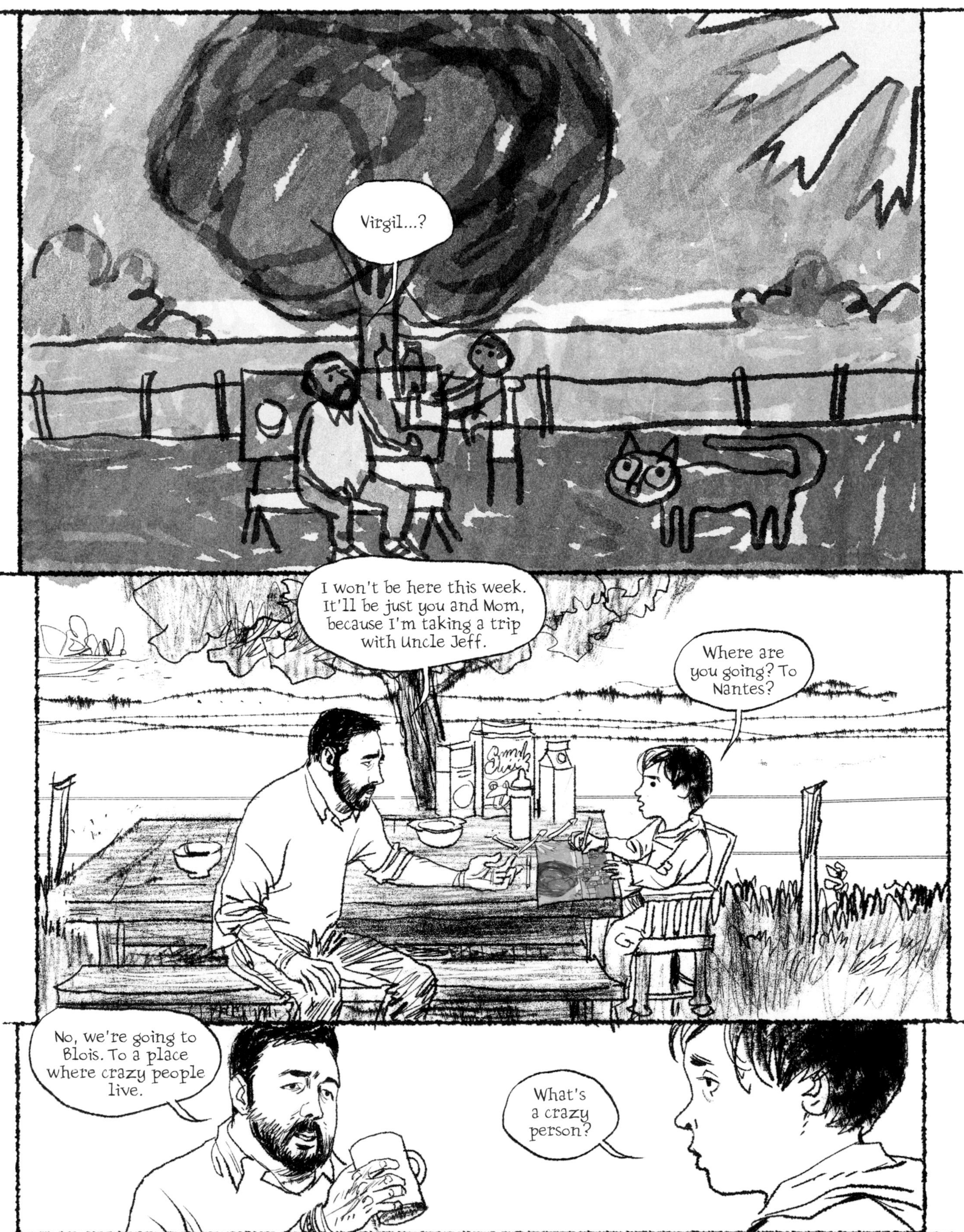
Virgil...?
I won't be here this week. It'll be just you and Mom, because I'm taking a trip with Uncle Jeff.
Where are you going? To Nantes?
No, we're going to Blois. To a place where crazy people live.
What's a crazy person?

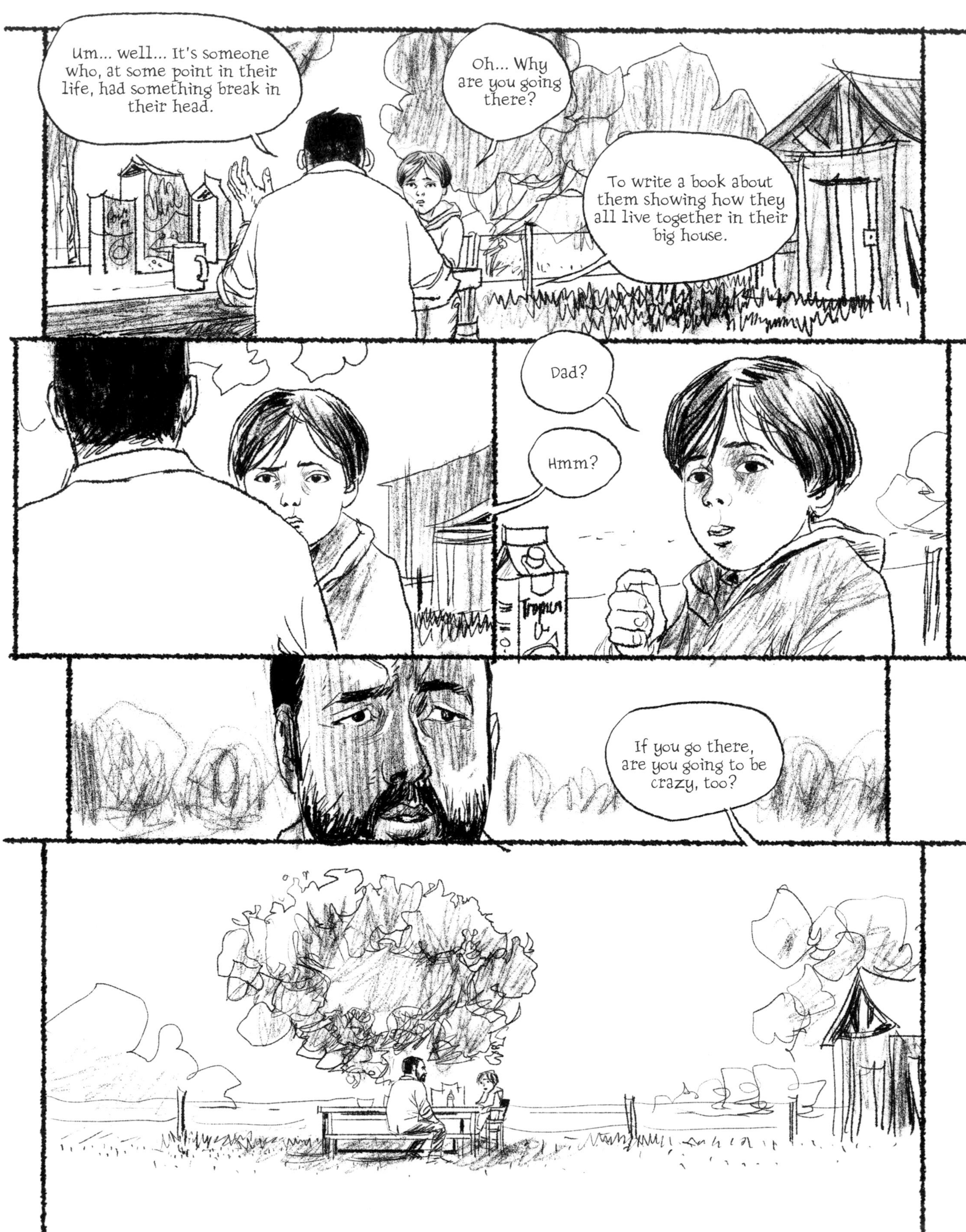
Um... well... It's someone who, at some point in their life, had something break in their head.
Oh... Why are you going there?
To write a book about them showing how they all live together in their big house.
Dad?
Hmm?
If you go there, are you going to be crazy, too?

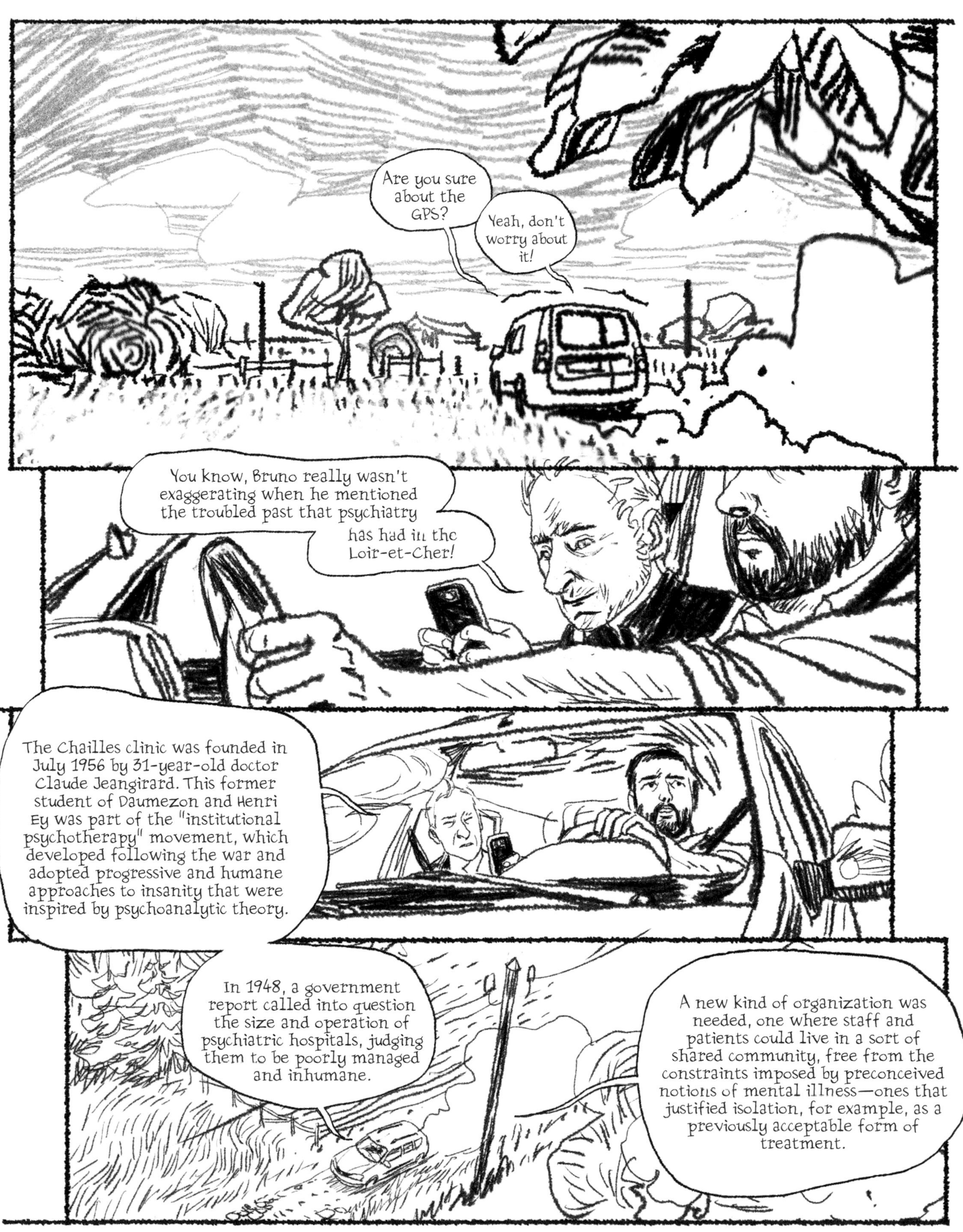

Are you sure about the GPS?
Yeah, don't worry about it!
You know, Bruno really wasn't exaggerating when he mentioned the troubled past that psychiatry has had in the Loir-et-Cher!
The Chailles clinic was founded in July 1956 by 31-year-old doctor Claude Jeangirard. This former student of Daumezon and Henri Ey was part of the "institutional psychotherapy" movement, which developed following the war and adopted progressive and humane approaches to insanity that were inspired by psychoanalytic theory.
In 1948, a government report called into question the size and operation of psychiatric hospitals, judging them to be poorly managed and inhumane.
A new kind of organization was needed, one where staff and patients could live in a sort of shared community, free from the constraints imposed by preconceived notions of mental illness—ones that justified isolation, for example, as a previously acceptable form of treatment.

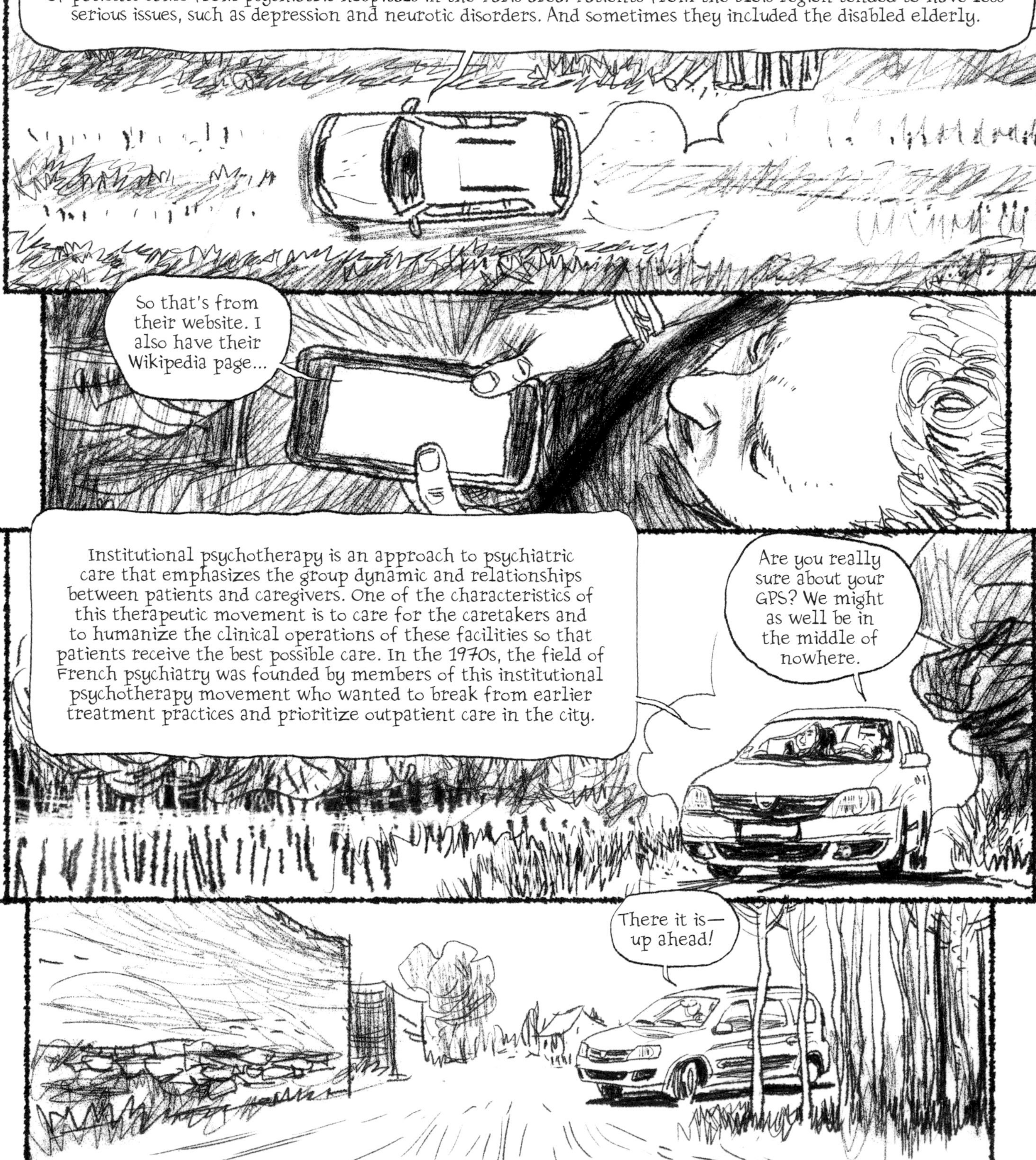
The reason for Chesnaie's creation, then, was to provide innovative care principally for the very sick in the public health system. This would usually involve long patient stays and—a fundamental principle of this kind of care—continuing the patients' care as their illness evolved. Different methods were used as deemed appropriate, including, but not limited to, hospitalization, in a holistic approach to patient care.
In June 1956, an agreement with the regional health insurance service in central France set the clinic's patient capacity at 45 at first, and then 60 within the next 2 years. The clinical staff was about 30 people, including 3 nurses, 1 social worker, 2 and then 3 doctors, and 1 part-time psychologist. In the beginning, a significant number of patients came from psychiatric hospitals in the Paris area. Patients from the Blois region tended to have less serious issues, such as depression and neurotic disorders. And sometimes they included the disabled elderly.
So that's from their website. I also have their Wikipedia page...
Institutional psychotherapy is an approach to psychiatric care that emphasizes the group dynamic and relationships between patients and caregivers. One of the characteristics of this therapeutic movement is to care for the caretakers and to humanize the clinical operations of these facilities so that patients receive the best possible care. In the 1970s, the field of French psychiatry was founded by members of this institutional psychotherapy movement who wanted to break from earlier treatment practices and prioritize outpatient care in the city.
Are you really sure about your GPS? We might as well be in the middle of nowhere.
There it is—up ahead!

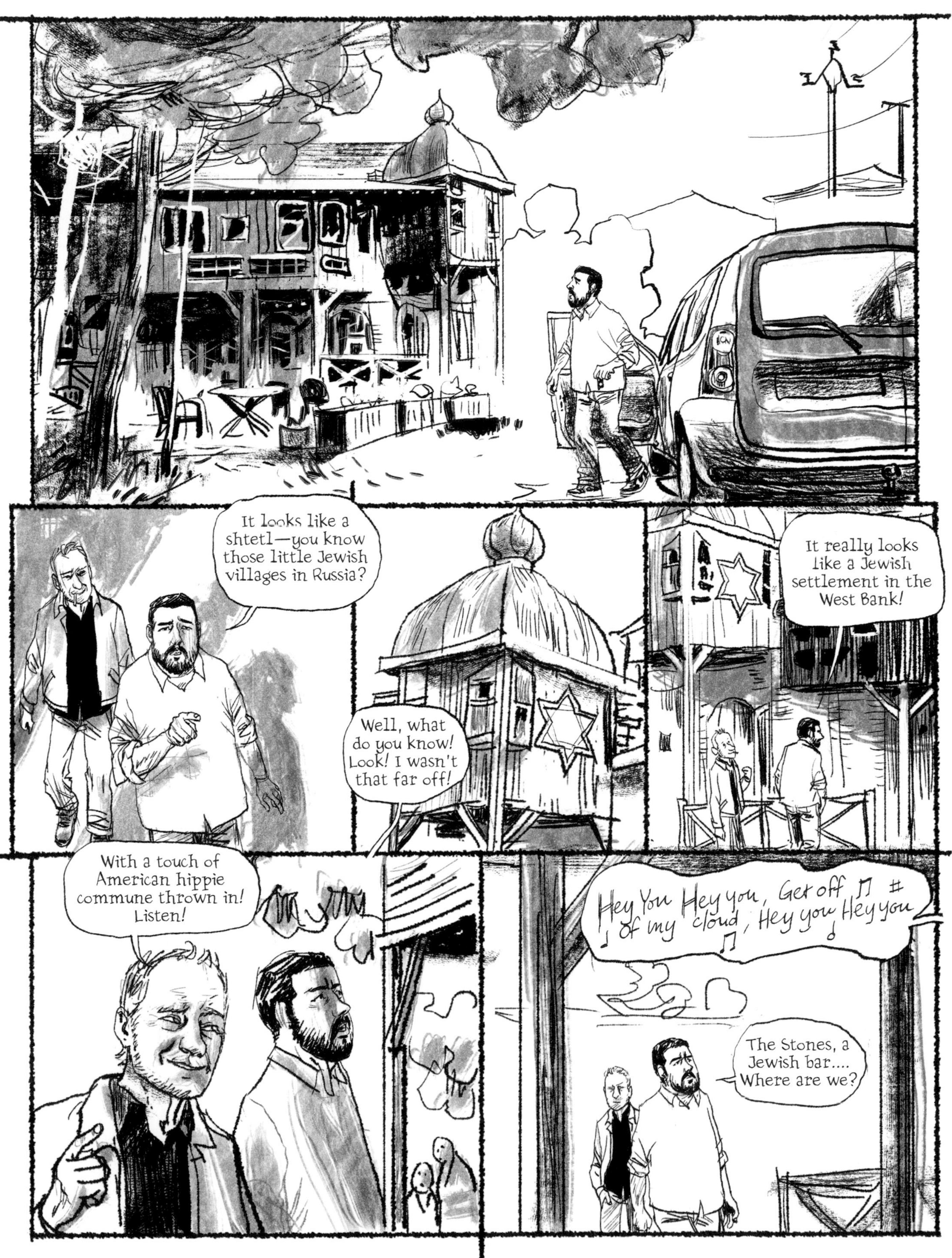
It looks like a shtetl—you know those little Jewish villages in Russia?
Well, what do you know! Look! I wasn't that far off!
It really looks like a Jewish settlement in the West Bank!
With a touch of American hippie commune thrown in! Listen!
Hey You Hey you, Get off of my cloud, Hey you Hey you
The Stones, a Jewish bar.... Where are we?

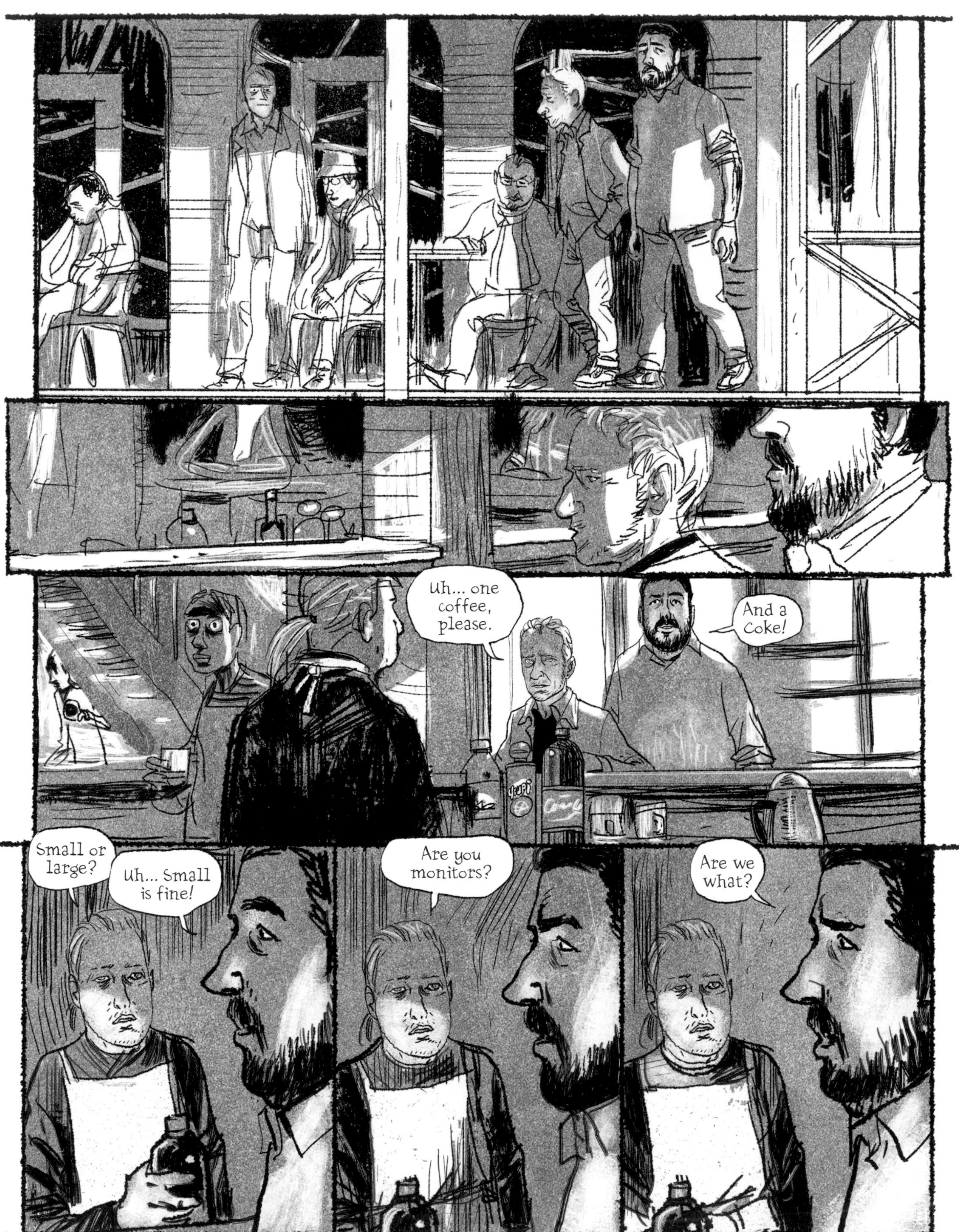
Uh... one coffee, please.
And a Coke!
Small or large?
Uh... Small is fine!
Are you monitors?
Are we what?

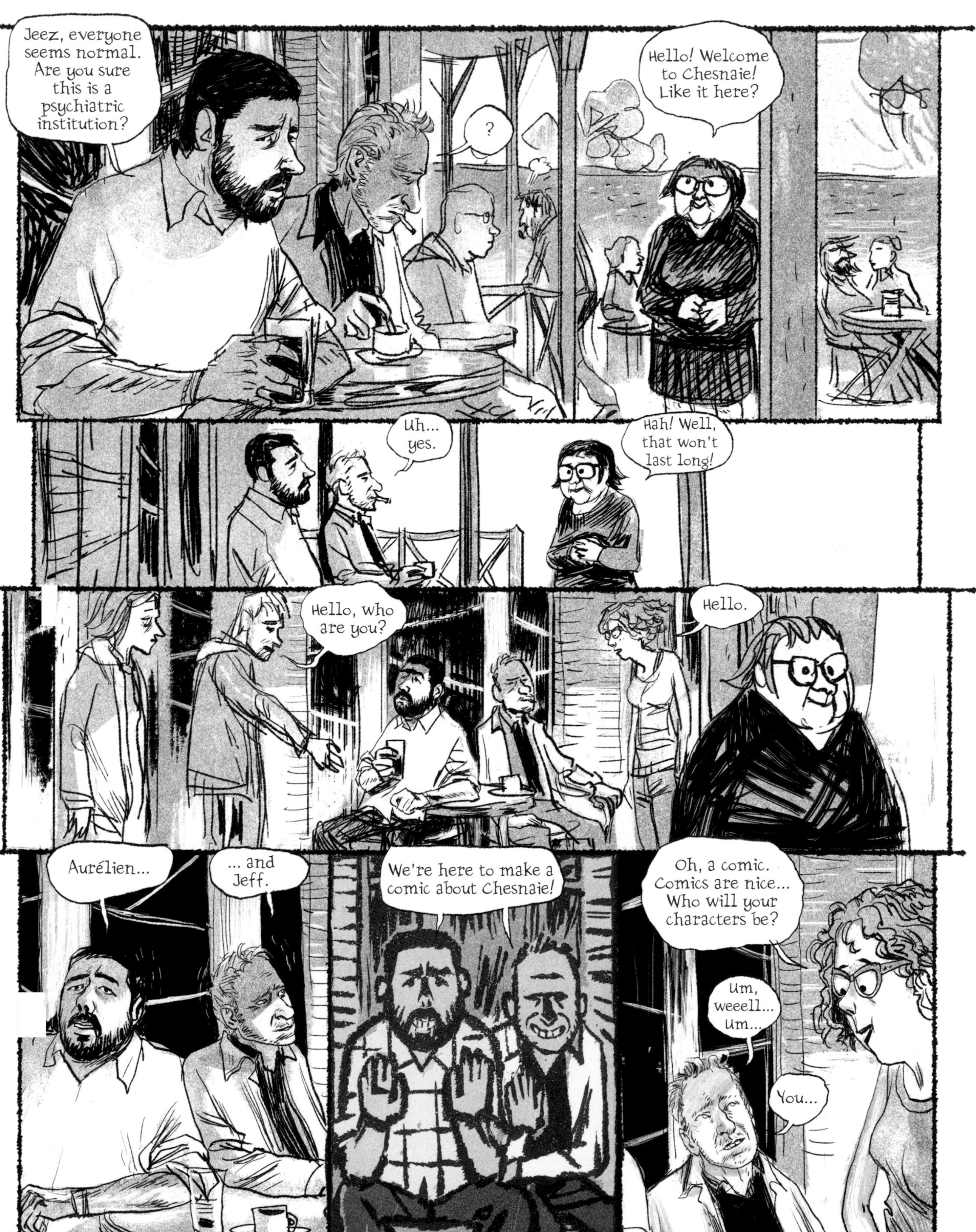
Jeez, everyone seems normal. Are you sure this is a psychiatric institution?
?
Hello! Welcome to Chesnaie! Like it here?
Uh... yes.
Hah! Well, that won't last long!
Hello, Who are you?
Hello.
Aurélien...
... and Jeff.
We're here to make a comic about Chesnaie!
Oh, a comic. Comics are nice... Who will your characters be?
Um, weeell... Um...
You...

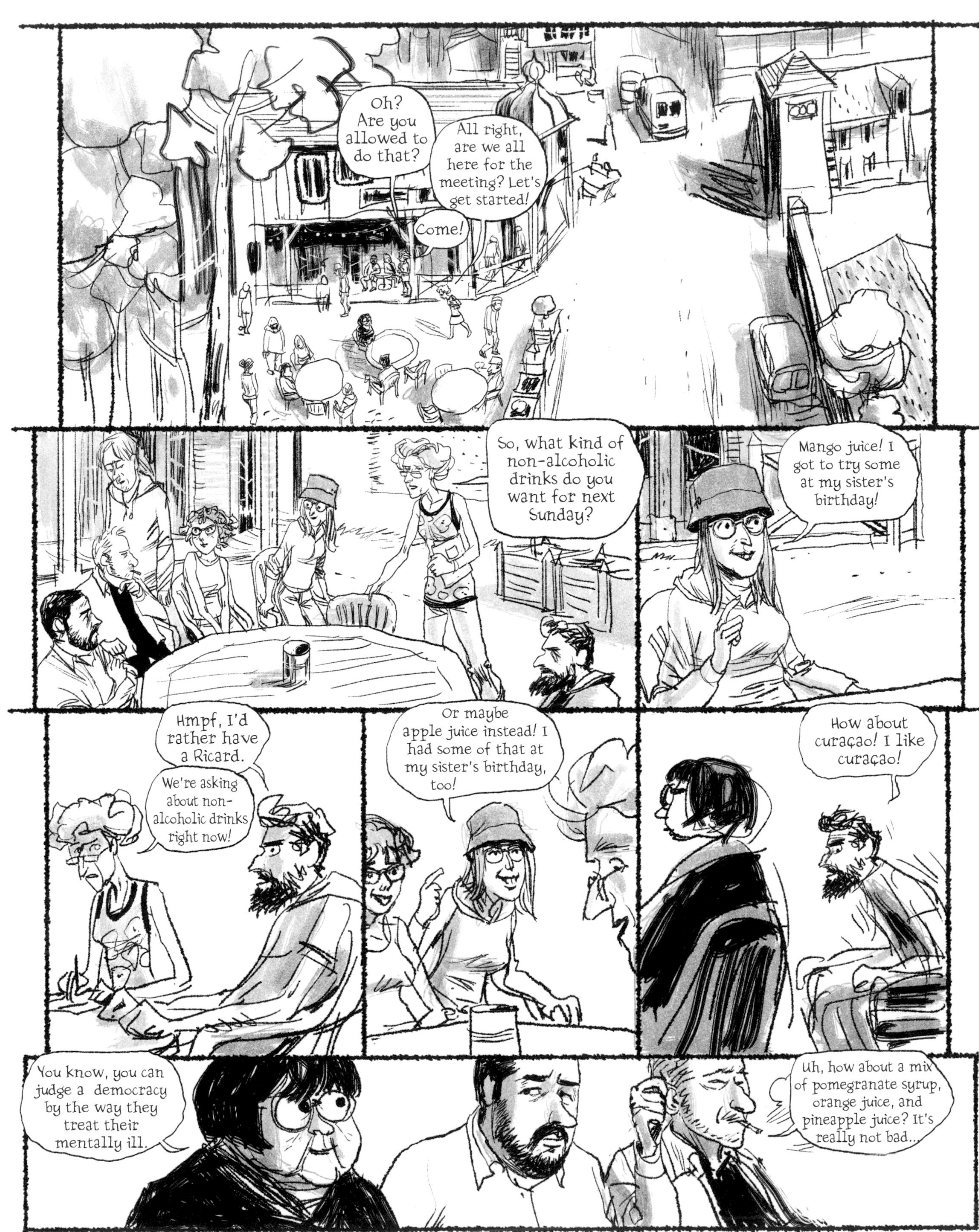
Oh? Are you allowed to do that?
All right, are we all here for the meeting? Let's get started!
Come!
So, what kind of non-alcoholic drinks do you want for next Sunday?
Mango juice! I got to try some at my sister's birthday!
Hmpf, I'd rather have a Ricard.
We're asking about non-alcoholic drinks right now!
Or maybe apple juice instead! I had some of that at my sister's birthday, too!
How about curaçao! I like curaçao!
You know, you can judge a democracy by the way they treat their mentally ill.
Uh, how about a mix of pomegranate syrup, orange juice, and pineapple juice? It's really not bad...

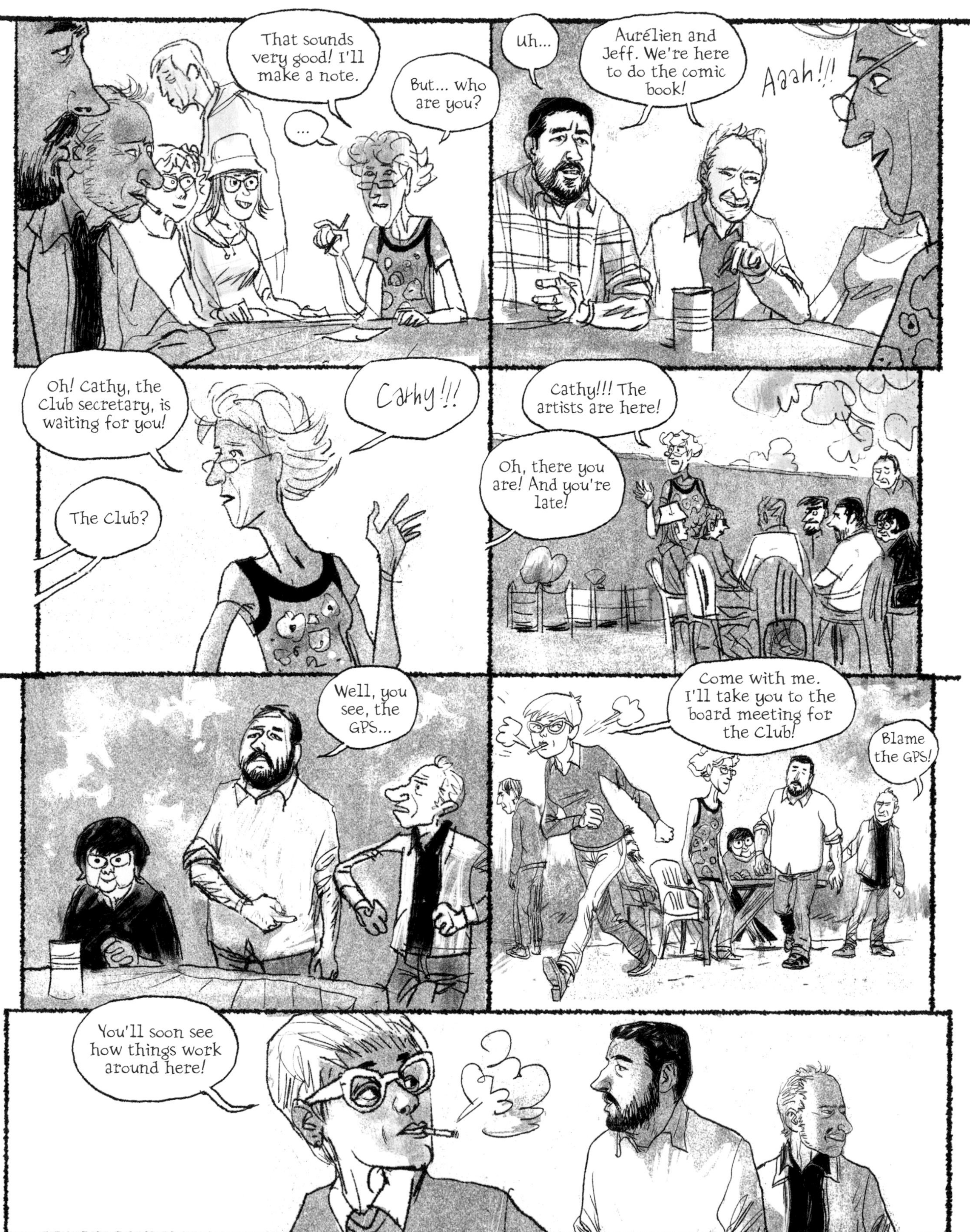
That sounds very good! I'll make a note.
...
But... who are you?
Uh...
Aurélien and Jeff. We're here to do the comic book!
Aaah!!!
Oh! Cathy, the Club secretary, is waiting for you!
Cathy!!!
The Club?
Cathy!!! The artists are here!
Oh, there you are! And you're late!
Well, you see, the GPS...
Come with me. I'll take you to the board meeting for the Club!
Blame the GPS!
You'll soon see how things work around here!

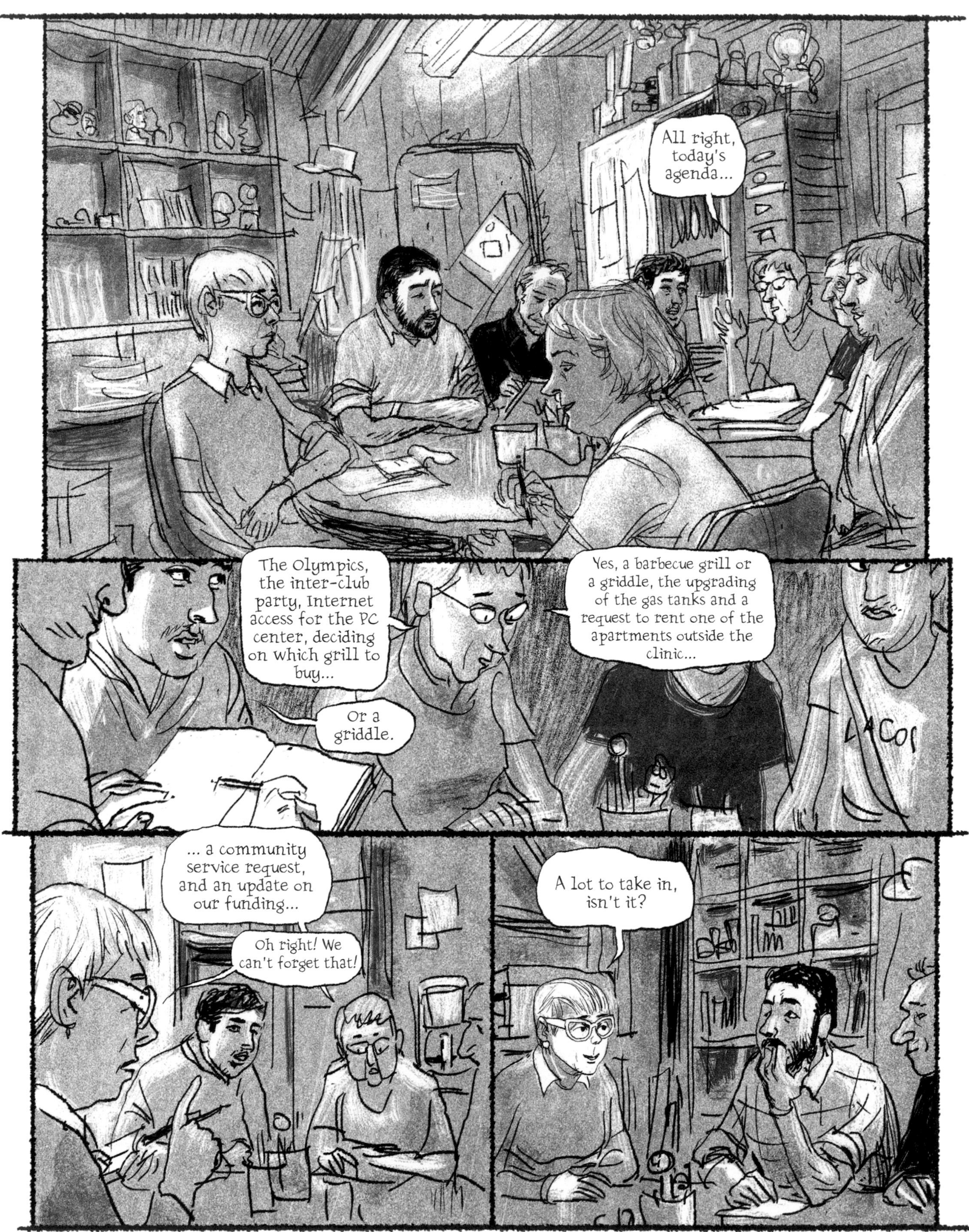
All right, today's agenda...
The Olympics, the inter-club party, Internet access for the PC center, deciding on which grill to buy...
Or a griddle.
Yes, a barbecue grill or a griddle, the upgrading of the gas tanks and a request to rent one of the apartments outside the clinic...
LACOI
... a community service request, and an update on our funding...
Oh right! We can't forget that!
A lot to take in, isn't it?

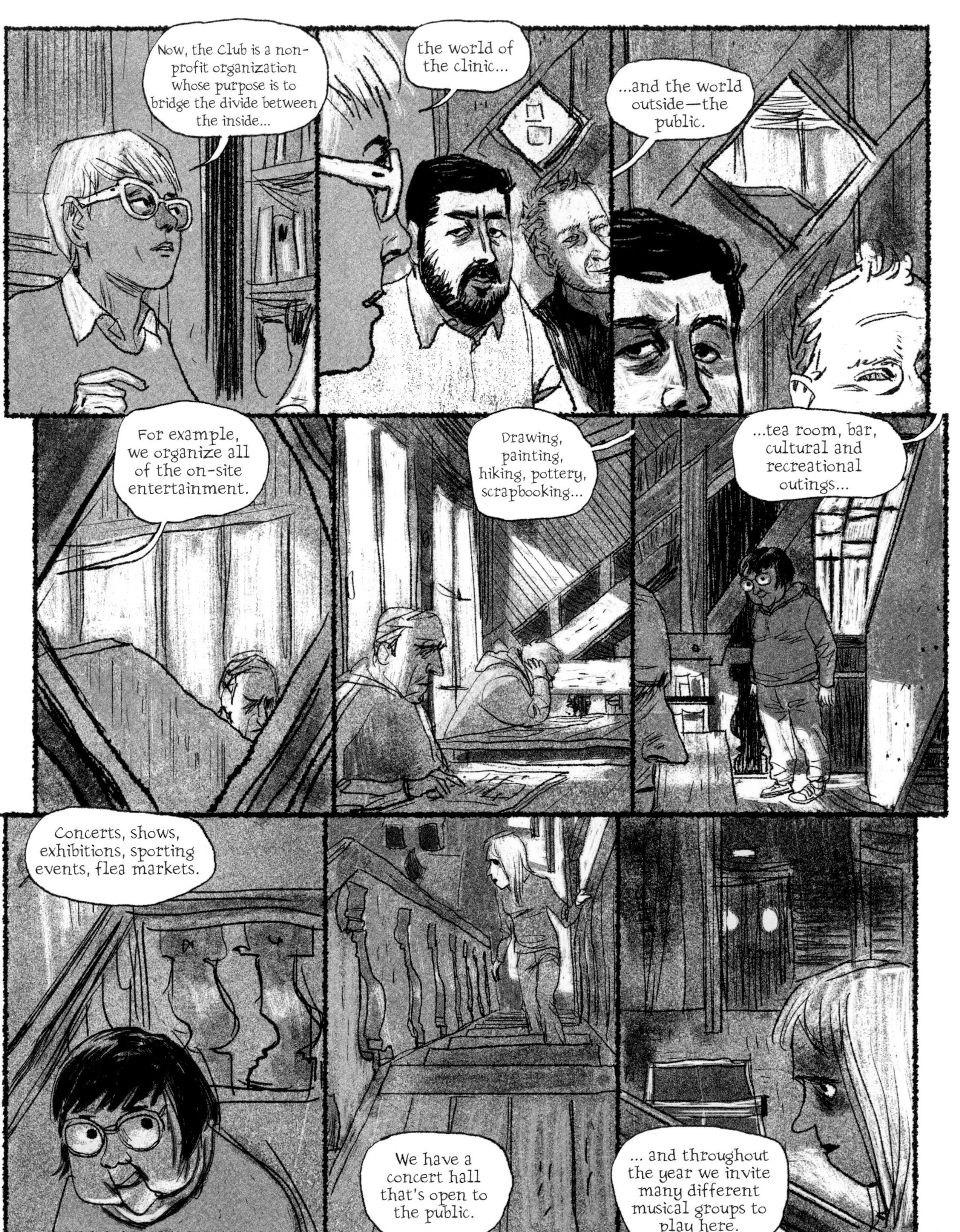
Now, the Club is a non-profit organization whose purpose is to bridge the divide between the inside...
the world of the clinic...
...and the world outside—the public.
For example, we organize all of the on-site entertainment.
Drawing, painting, hiking, pottery, scrapbooking...
...tea room, bar, cultural and recreational outings...
Concerts, shows, exhibitions, sporting events, flea markets.
We have a concert hall that's open to the public.
... and throughout the year we invite many different musical groups to play here.

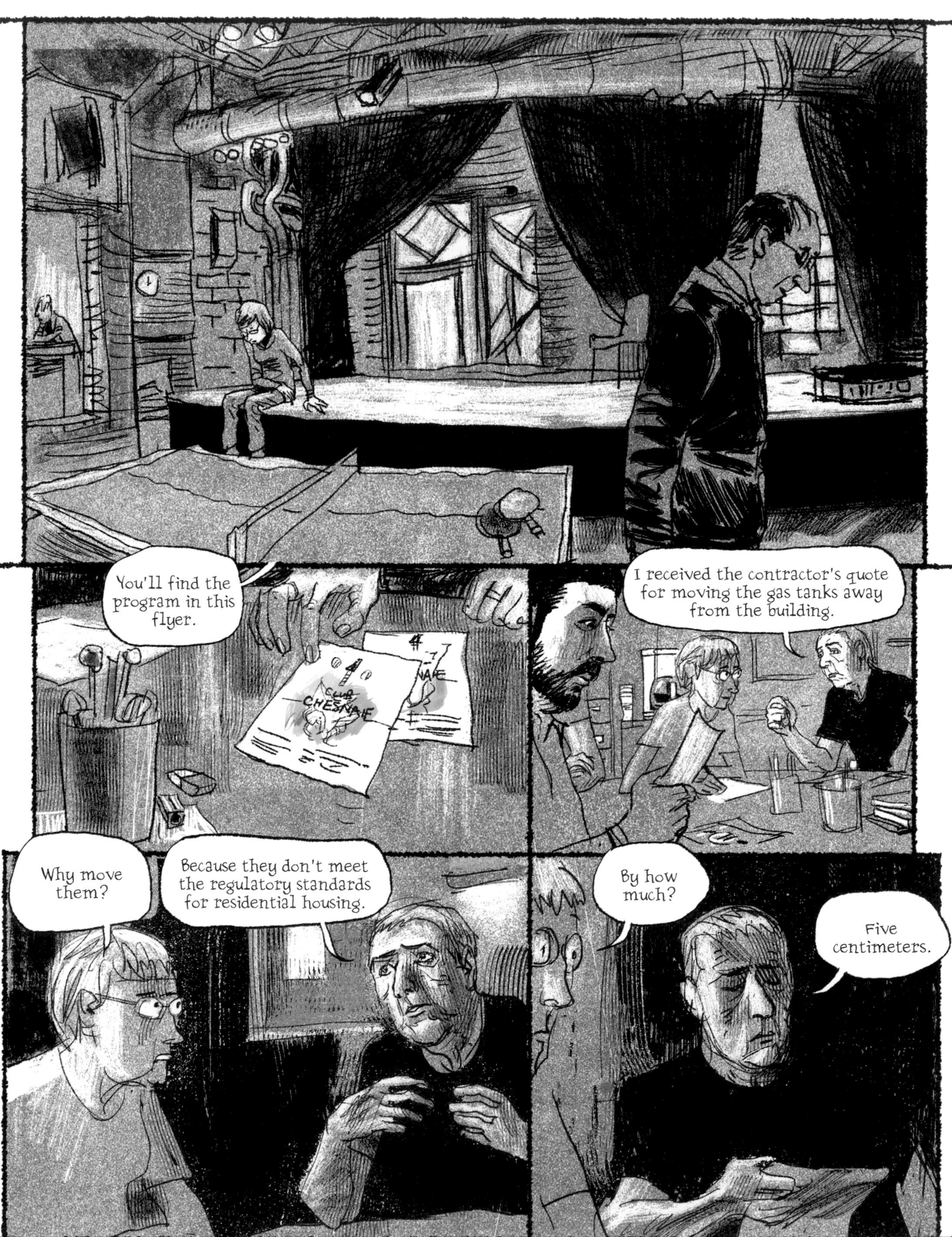
You'll find the program in this flyer.
CLUB CHESNAIE
I received the contractor's quote for moving the gas tanks away from the building.
Why move them?
Because they don't meet the regulatory standards for residential housing.
By how much?
Five centimeters.

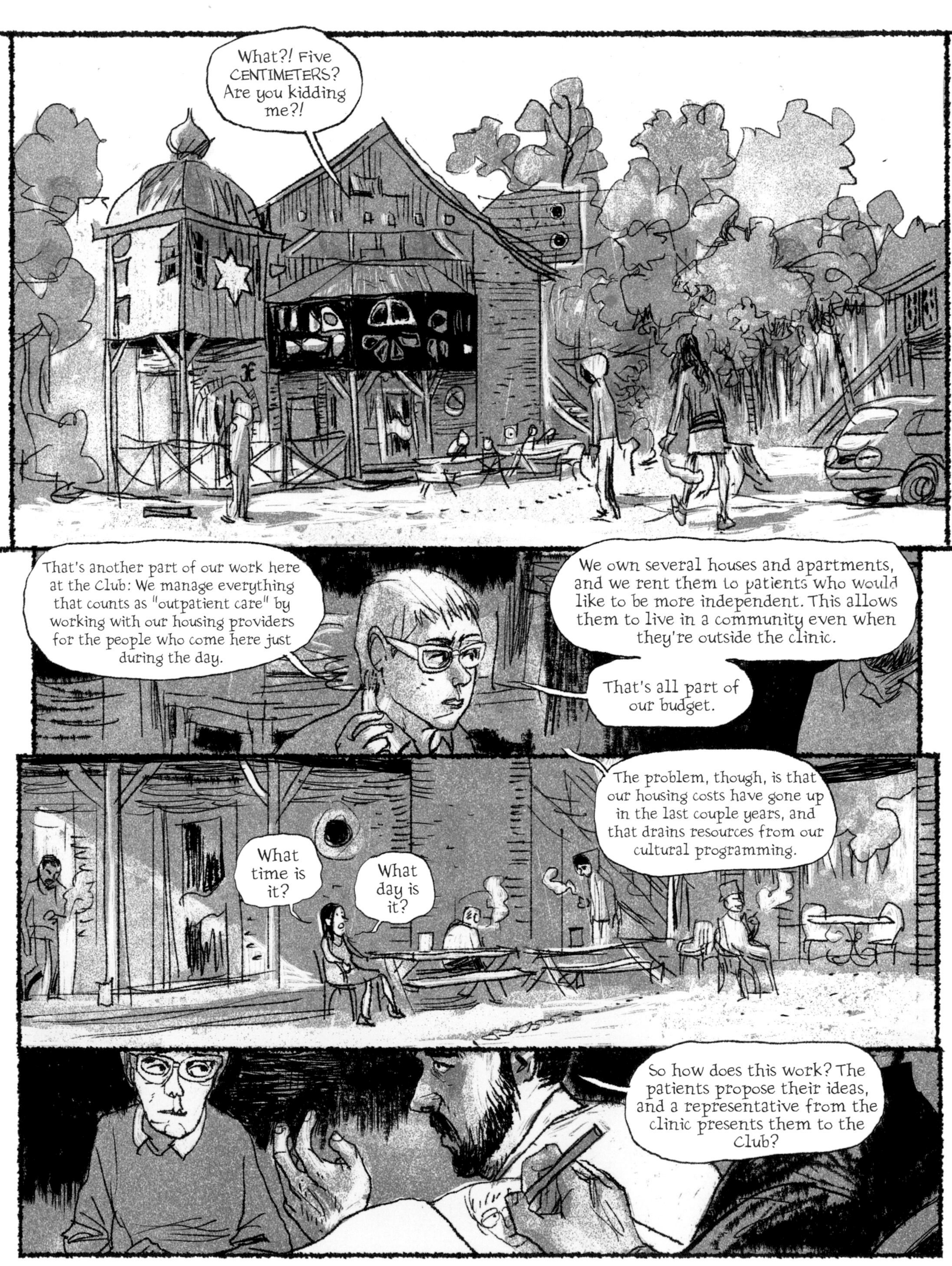
What?! Five CENTIMETERS? Are you kidding me?!
That's another part of our work here at the Club: We manage everything that counts as "outpatient care" by working with our housing providers for the people who come here just during the day.
We own several houses and apartments, and we rent them to patients who would like to be more independent. This allows them to live in a community even when they're outside the clinic.
That's all part of our budget.
The problem, though, is that our housing costs have gone up in the last couple years, and that drains resources from our cultural programming.
What time is it?
What day is it?
So how does this work? The patients propose their ideas, and a representative from the clinic presents them to the Club?

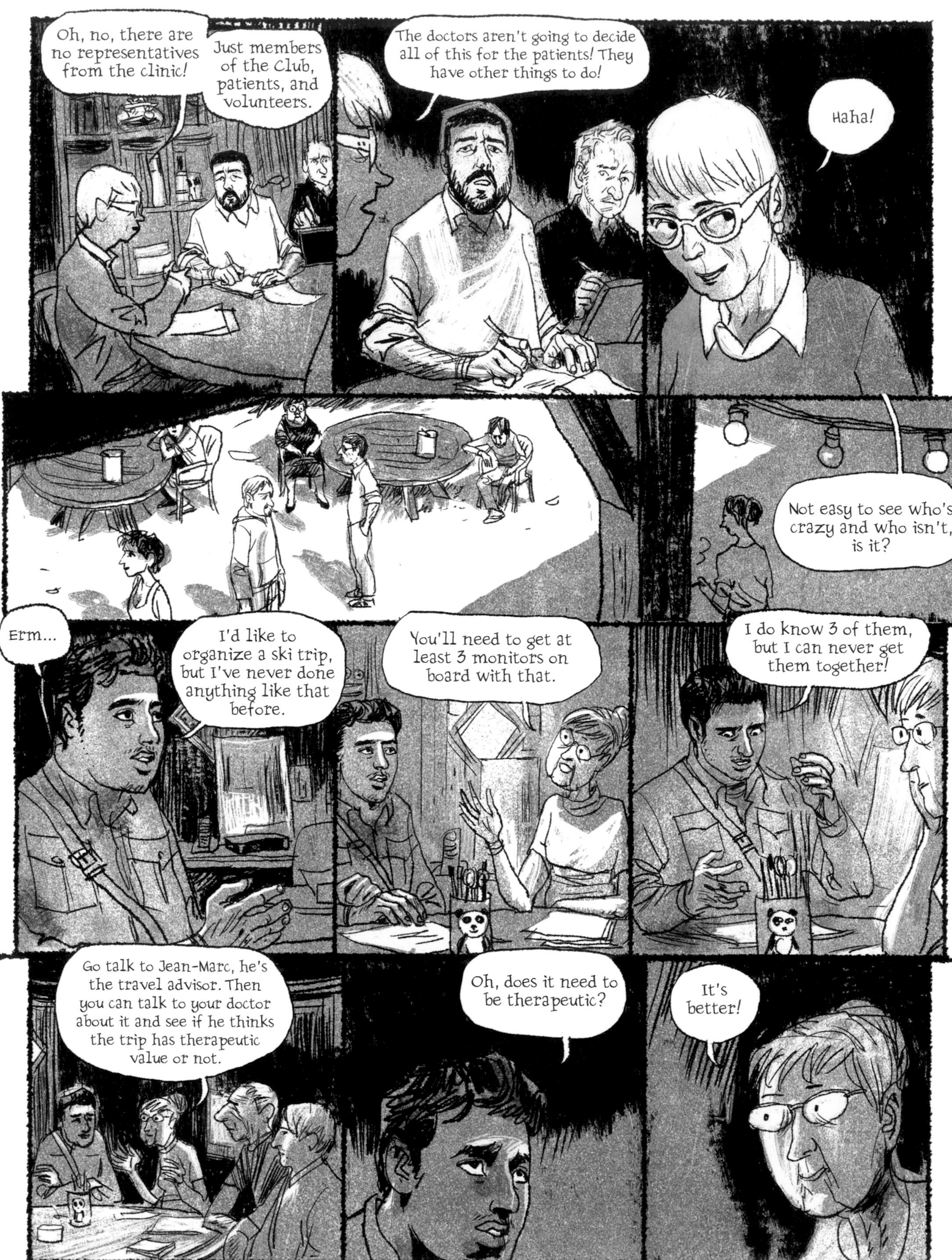
Oh, no, there are no representatives from the clinic!
Just members of the Club, patients, and volunteers.
The doctors aren't going to decide all of this for the patients! They have other things to do!
Haha!
Not easy to see who's crazy and who isn't, is it?
Erm...
I'd like to organize a ski trip, but I've never done anything like that before.
You'll need to get at least 3 monitors on board with that.
I do know 3 of them, but I can never get them together!
Go talk to Jean-Marc, he's the travel advisor. Then you can talk to your doctor about it and see if he thinks the trip has therapeutic value or not.
Oh, does it need to be therapeutic?
It's better!

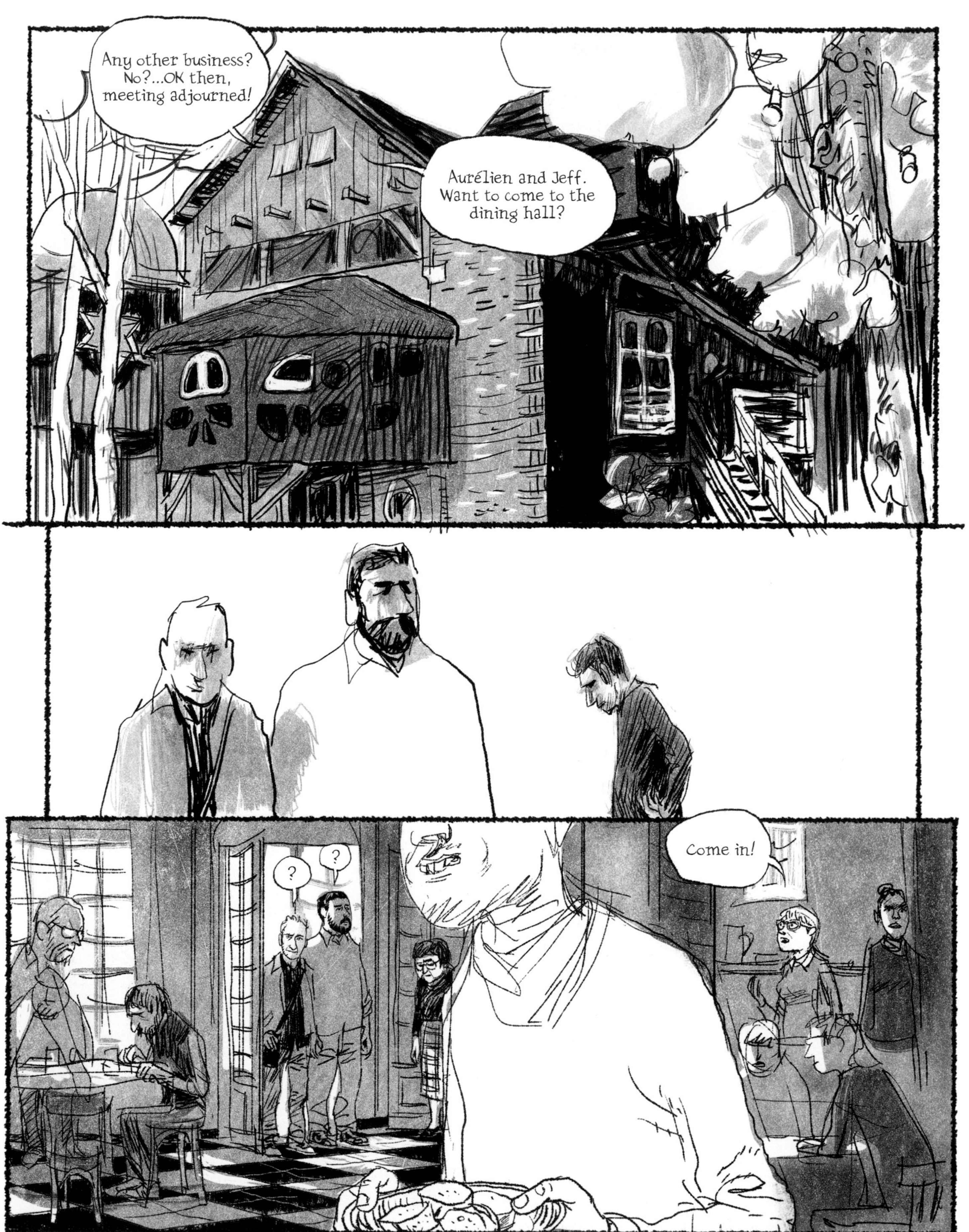
Any other business? No?...OK then, meeting adjourned!
Aurélien and Jeff. Want to come to the dining hall?
?
?
Come in!

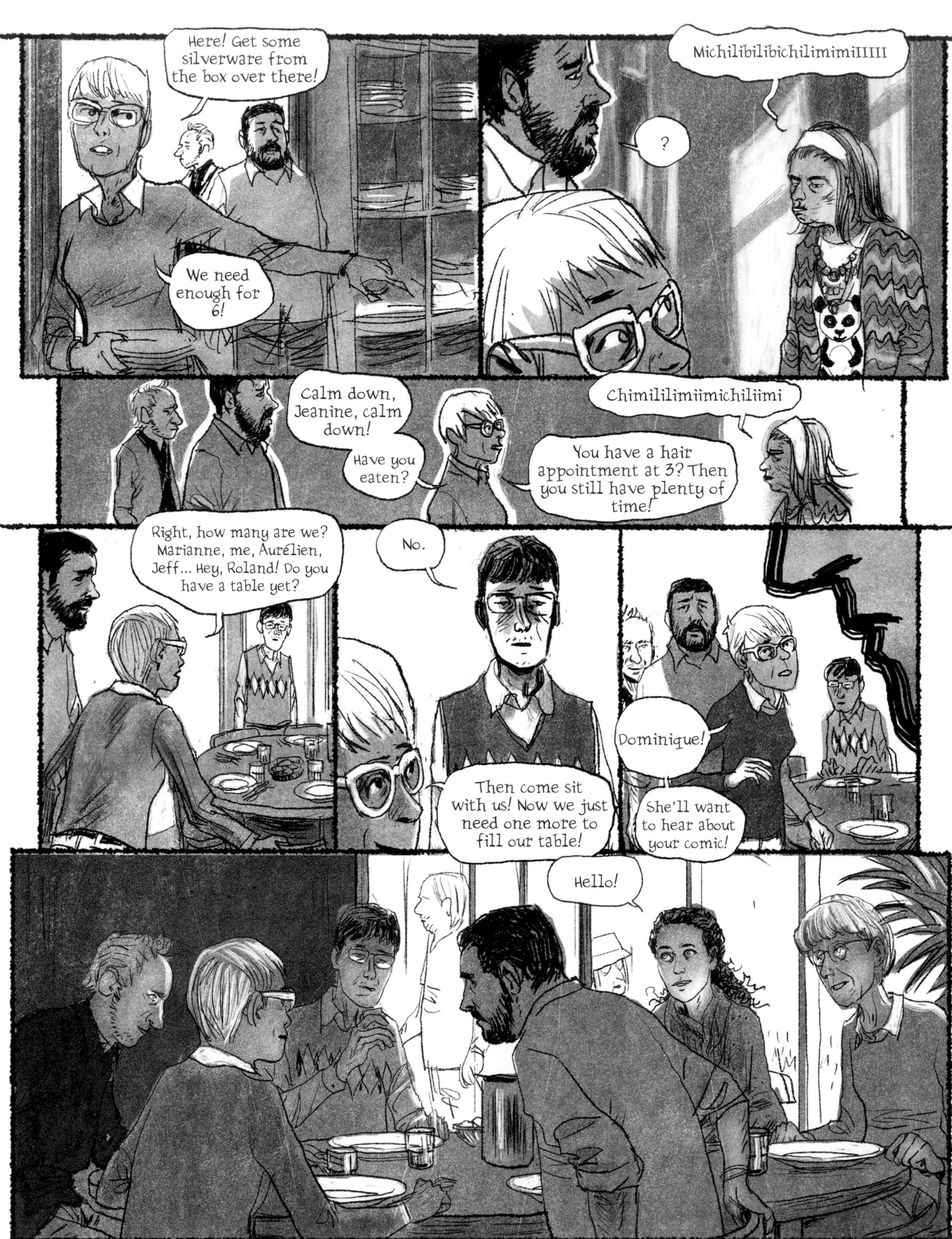
Here! Get some silverware from the box over there!
We need enough for 6!
MichilibilibichilimimiIIIII
?
Calm down, Jeanine, calm down!
Have you eaten?
Chimililimiimichiliimi
You have a hair appointment at 3? Then you still have plenty of time!
Right, how many are we? Marianne, me, Aurélien, Jeff... Hey, Roland! Do you have a table yet?
No.
Then come sit with us! Now we just need one more to fill our table!
Dominique!
She'll want to hear about your comic!
Hello!

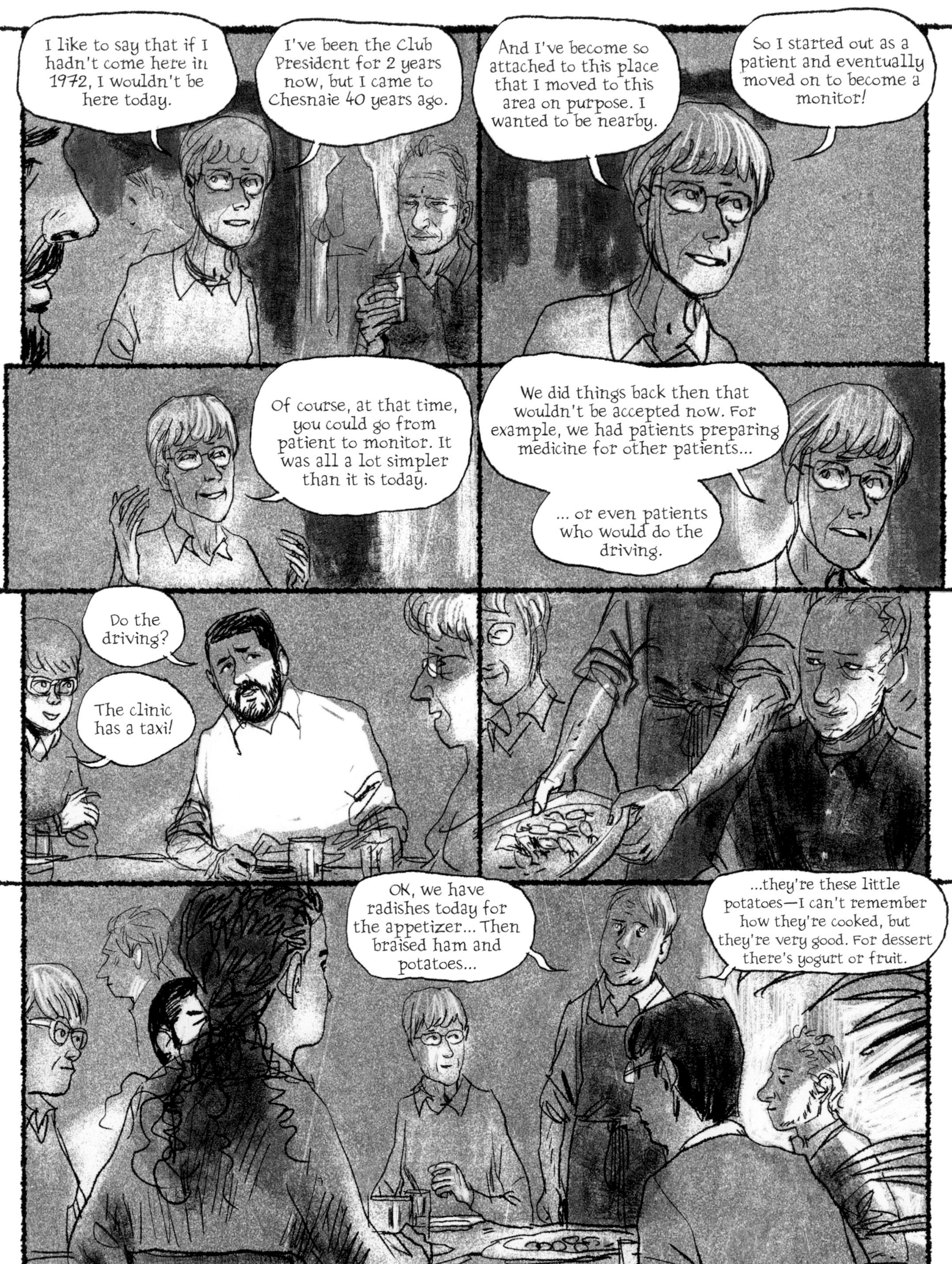
I like to say that if I hadn't come here in 1972, I wouldn't be here today.
I've been the Club President for 2 years now, but I came to Chesnaie 40 years ago.
And I've become so attached to this place that I moved to this area on purpose. I wanted to be nearby.
So I started out as a patient and eventually moved on to become a monitor!
Of course, at that time, you could go from patient to monitor. It was all a lot simpler than it is today.
We did things back then that wouldn't be accepted now. For example, we had patients preparing medicine for other patients...
... or even patients who would do the driving.
Do the driving?
The clinic has a taxi!
OK, we have radishes today for the appetizer... Then braised ham and potatoes...
...they're these little potatoes—I can't remember how they're cooked, but they're very good. For dessert there's yogurt or fruit.

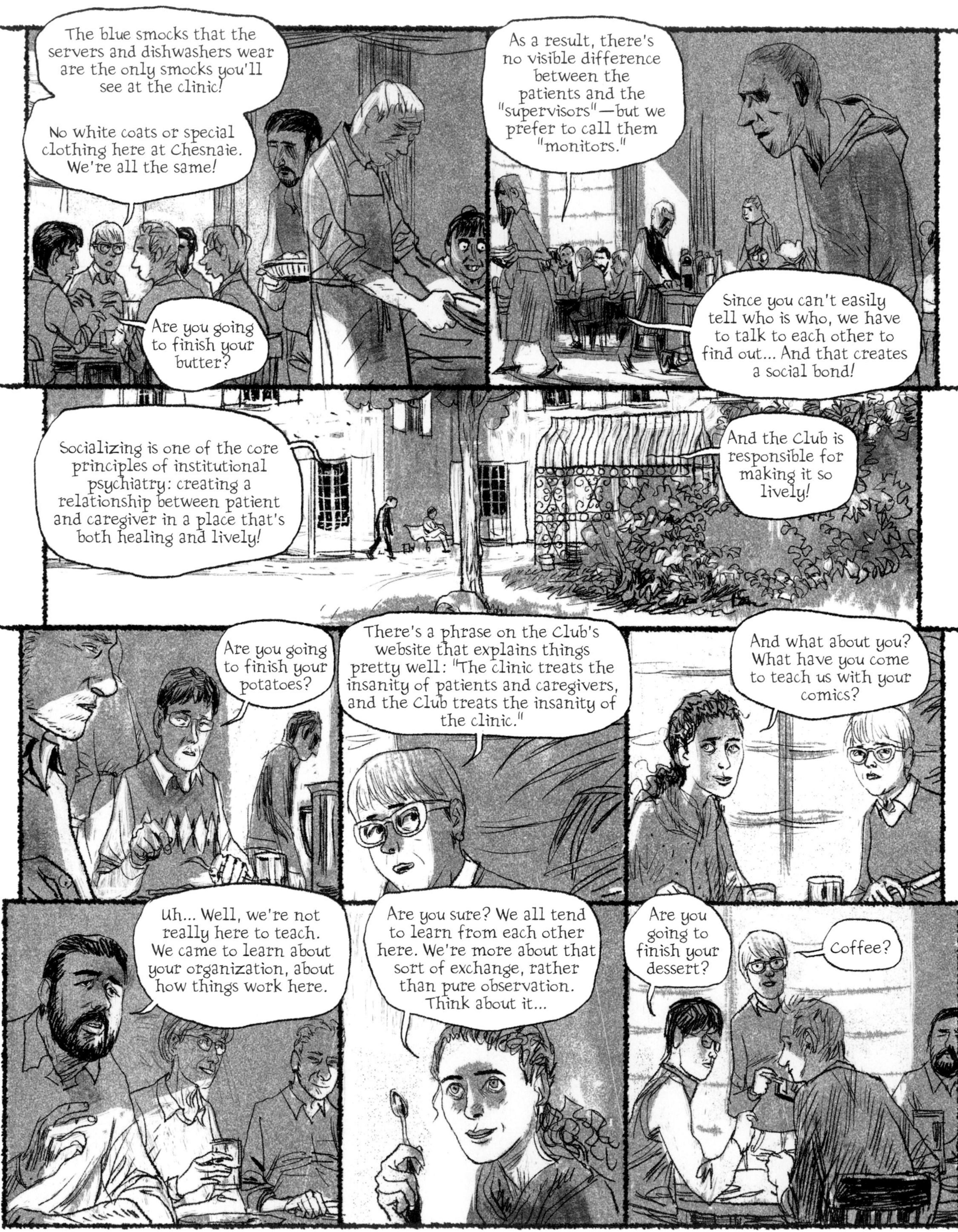
The blue smocks that the servers and dishwashers wear are the only smocks you'll see at the clinic!
No white coats or special clothing here at Chesnaie. We're all the same!
Are you going to finish your butter?
As a result, there's no visible difference between the patients and the "supervisors"—but we prefer to call them "monitors."
Since you can't easily tell who is who, we have to talk to each other to find out... And that creates a social bond!
Socializing is one of the core principles of institutional psychiatry: creating a relationship between patient and caregiver in a place that's both healing and lively!
And the Club is responsible for making it so lively!
Are you going to finish your potatoes?
There's a phrase on the Club's website that explains things pretty well: "The clinic treats the insanity of patients and caregivers, and the Club treats the insanity of the clinic."
And what about you? What have you come to teach us with your comics?
Uh... Well, we're not really here to teach. We came to learn about your organization, about how things work here.
Are you sure? We all tend to learn from each other here. We're more about that sort of exchange, rather than pure observation. Think about it...
Are you going to finish your dessert?
Coffee?

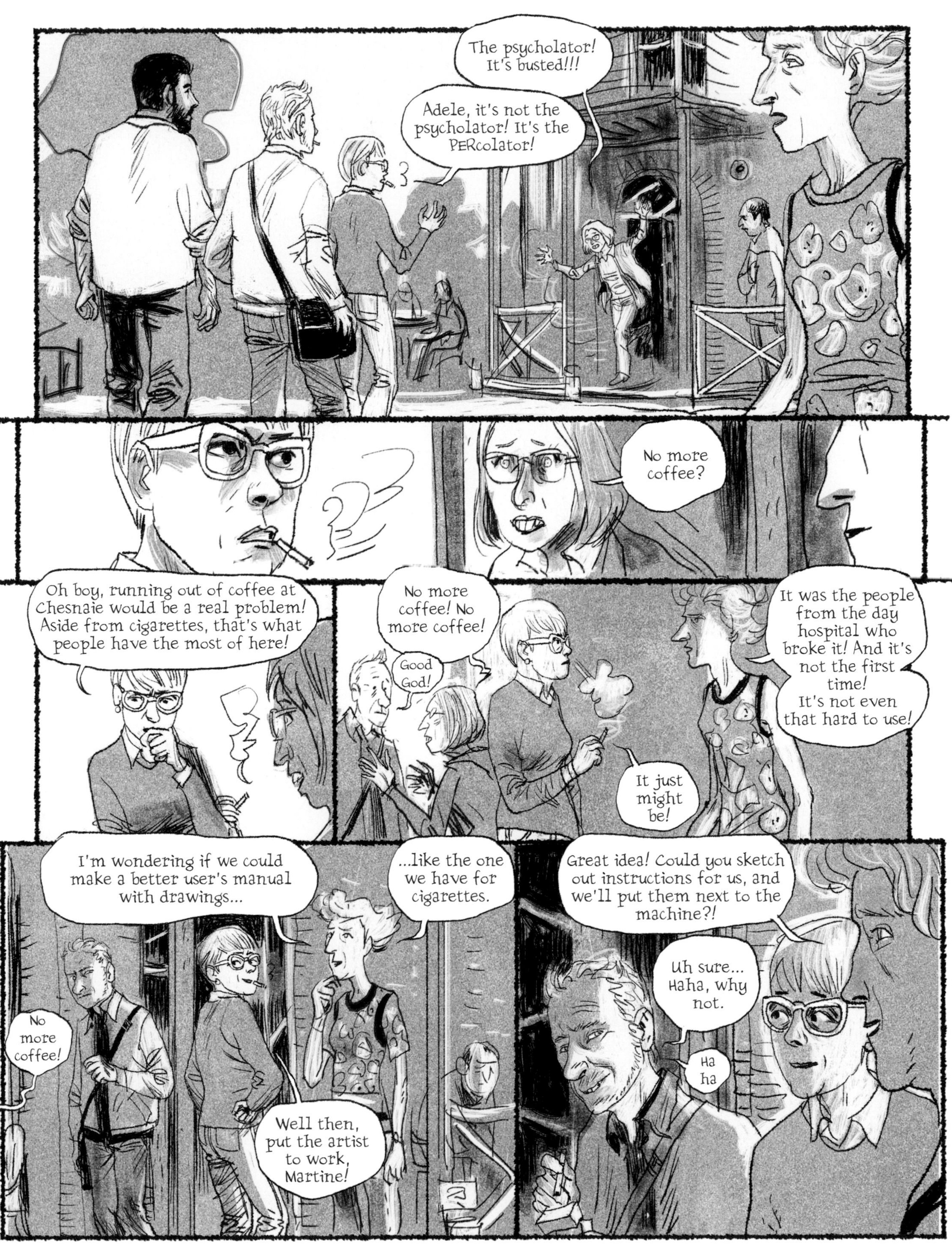
The psycholator! It's busted!!!
Adele, it's not the psycholator! It's the PERcolator!
No more coffee?
Oh boy, running out of coffee at Chesnaie would be a real problem! Aside from cigarettes, that's what people have the most of here!
No more coffee! No more coffee!
Good God!
It was the people from the day hospital who broke it! And it's not the first time! It's not even that hard to use!
It just might be!
I'm wondering if we could make a better user's manual with drawings...
...like the one we have for cigarettes.
No more coffee!
Well then, put the artist to work, Martine!
Great idea! Could you sketch out instructions for us, and we'll put them next to the machine?!
Uh sure... Haha, why not.
Ha ha

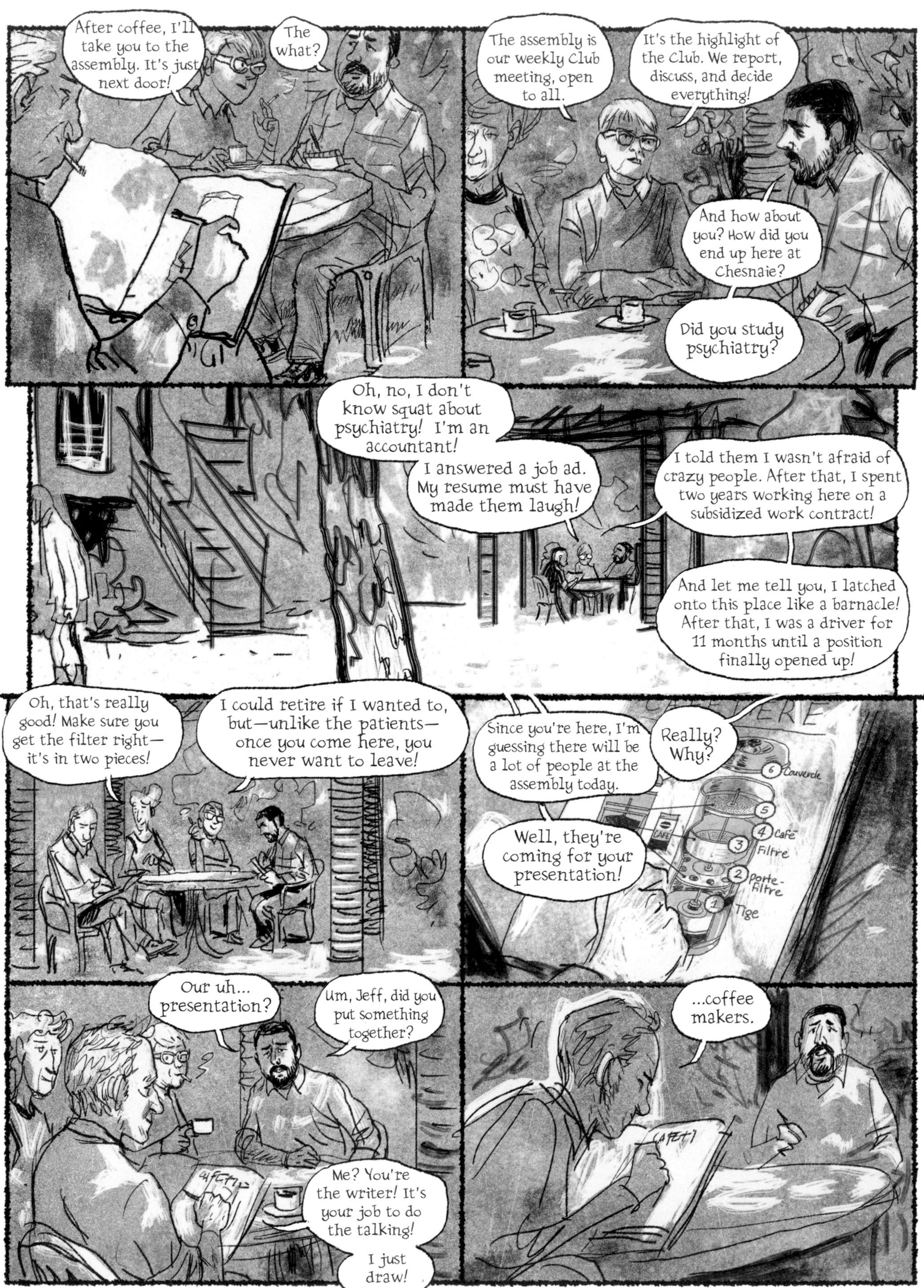
After coffee, I'll take you to the assembly. It's just next door!
The what?
The assembly is our weekly Club meeting, open to all.
It's the highlight of the Club. We report, discuss, and decide everything!
And how about you? How did you end up here at Chesnaie?
Did you study psychiatry?
Oh, no, I don't know squat about psychiatry! I'm an accountant!
I answered a job ad. My resume must have made them laugh!
I told them I wasn't afraid of crazy people. After that, I spent two years working here on a subsidized work contract!
And let me tell you, I latched onto this place like a barnacle! After that, I was a driver for 11 months until a position finally opened up!
Oh, that's really good! Make sure you get the filter right—it's in two pieces!
I could retire if I wanted to, but—unlike the patients—once you come here, you never want to leave!
Since you're here, I'm guessing there will be a lot of people at the assembly today.
Really? Why?
Well, they're coming for your presentation!
6 Couvercle
5
4 Café
3 Filtre
2 Porte-filtre
1 Tige
Our uh... presentation?
Um, Jeff, did you put something together?
Me? You're the writer! It's your job to do the talking!
I just draw!
...coffee makers.

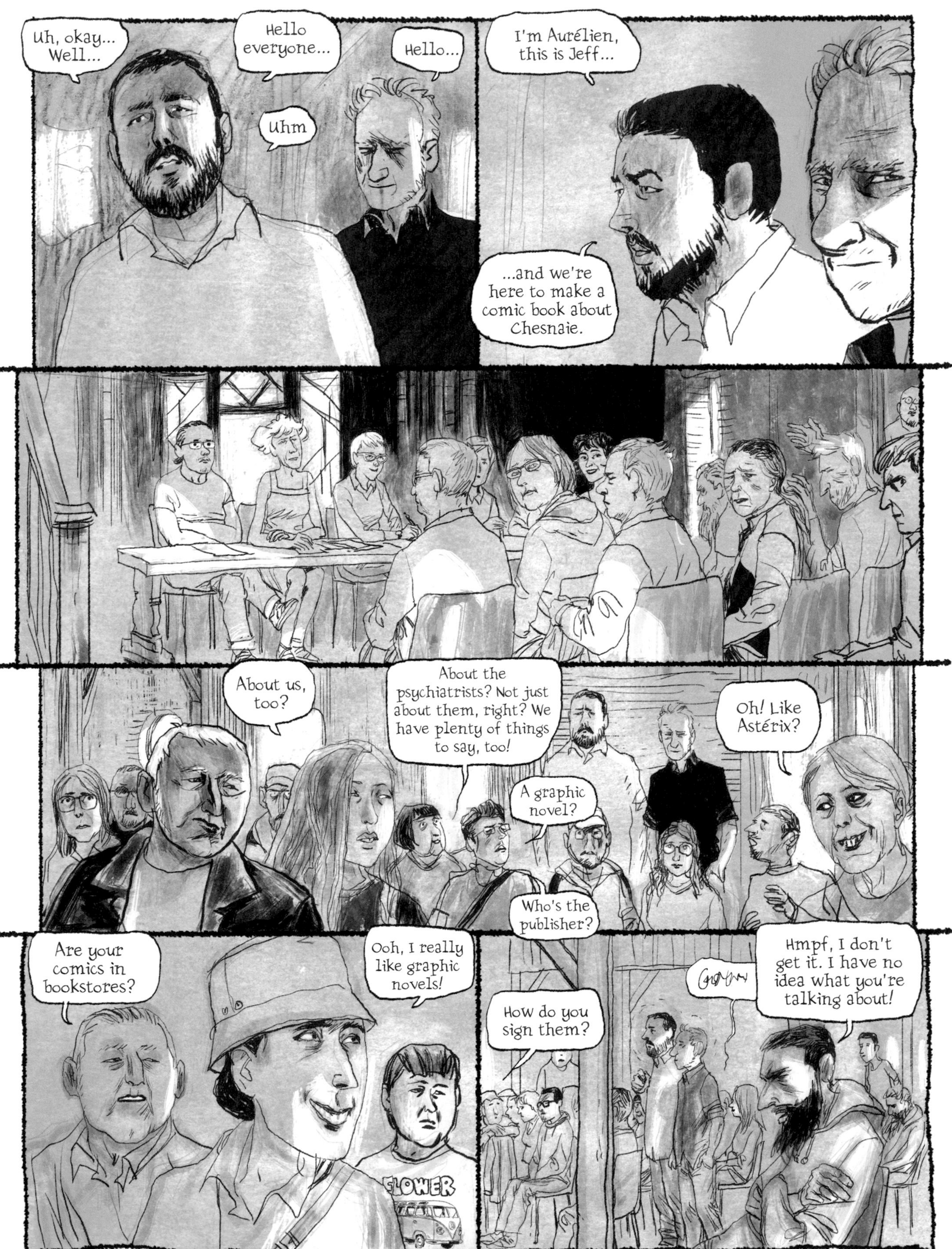
Uh, okay... Well...
Hello everyone...
Hello...
Uhm
I'm Aurélien, this is Jeff...
...and we're here to make a comic book about Chesnaie.
About us, too?
About the psychiatrists? Not just about them, right? We have plenty of things to say, too!
Oh! Like Astérix?
A graphic novel?
Who's the publisher?
Are your comics in bookstores?
Ooh, I really like graphic novels!
How do you sign them?
Hmpf, I don't get it. I have no idea what you're talking about!
FLOWER

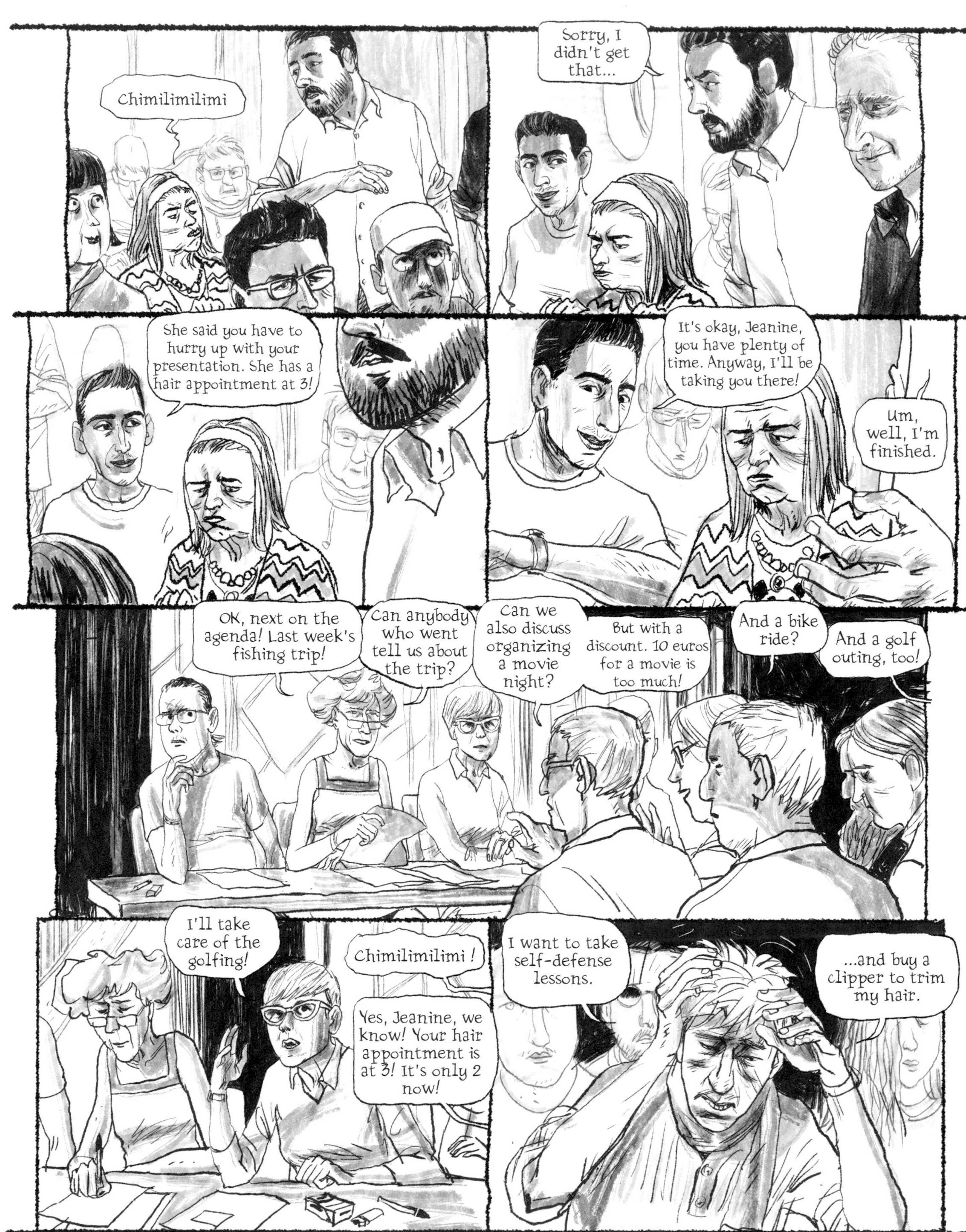
Chimilimilimi
Sorry, I didn't get that...
She said you have to hurry up with your presentation. She has a hair appointment at 3!
It's okay, Jeanine, you have plenty of time. Anyway, I'll be taking you there!
Um, well, I'm finished.
OK, next on the agenda! Last week's fishing trip!
Can anybody who went tell us about the trip?
Can we also discuss organizing a movie night?
But with a discount. 10 euros for a movie is too much!
And a bike ride?
And a golf outing, too!
I'll take care of the golfing!
Chimilimilimi !
Yes, Jeanine, we know! Your hair appointment is at 3! It's only 2 now!
I want to take self-defense lessons.
...and buy a clipper to trim my hair.

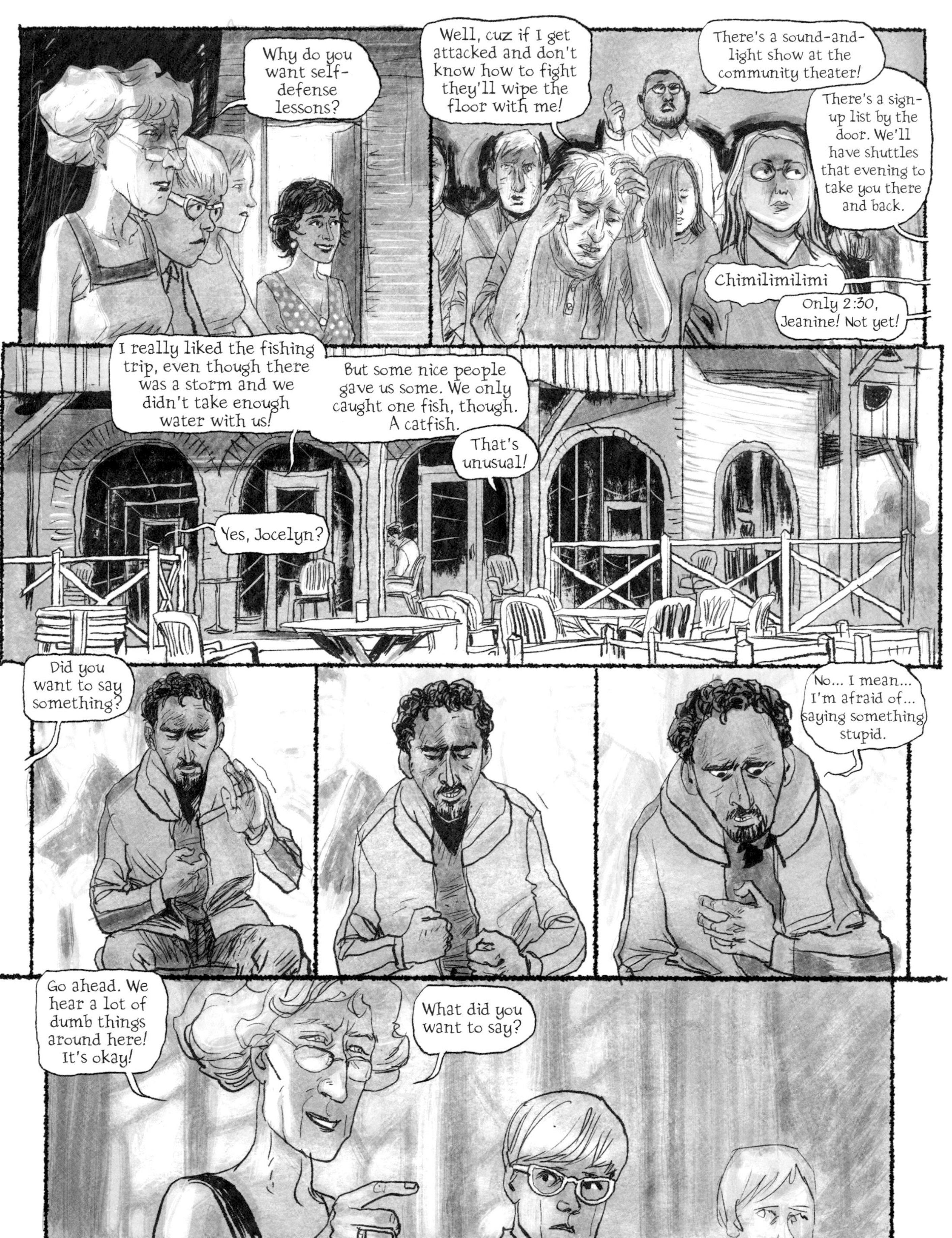
Why do you want self-defense lessons?
Well, cuz if I get attacked and don't know how to fight they'll wipe the floor with me!
There's a sound-and-light show at the community theater!
There's a sign-up list by the door. We'll have shuttles that evening to take you there and back.
Chimilimilimi
Only 2:30, Jeanine! Not yet!
I really liked the fishing trip, even though there was a storm and we didn't take enough water with us!
But some nice people gave us some. We only caught one fish, though. A catfish.
That's unusual!
Yes, Jocelyn?
Did you want to say something?
No... I mean... I'm afraid of... saying something stupid.
Go ahead. We hear a lot of dumb things around here! It's okay!
What did you want to say?

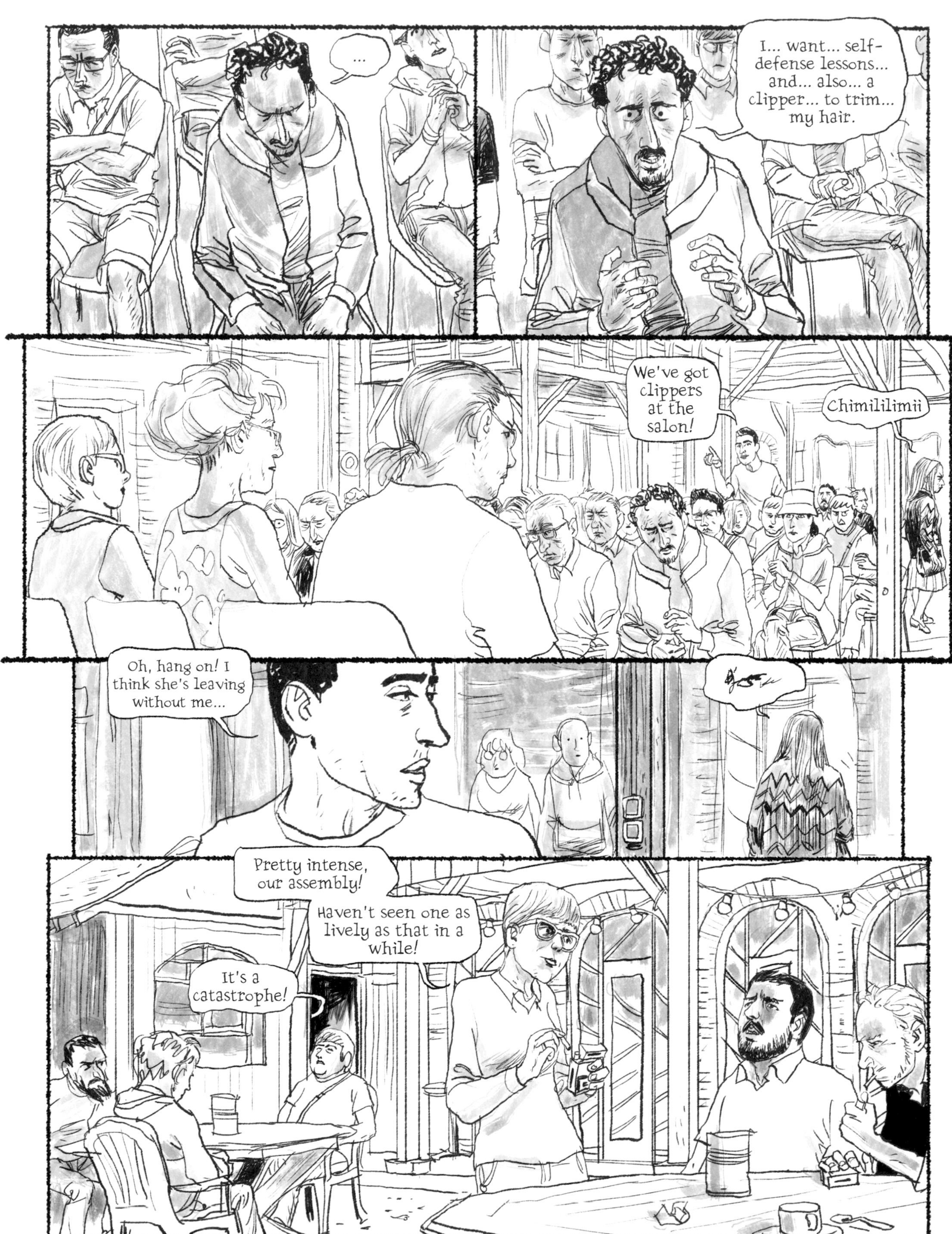
...
I... want... self-defense lessons... and... also... a clipper... to trim... my hair.
We've got clippers at the salon!
Chimililimii
Oh, hang on! I think she's leaving without me...
Pretty intense, our assembly!
Haven't seen one as lively as that in a while!
It's a catastrophe!

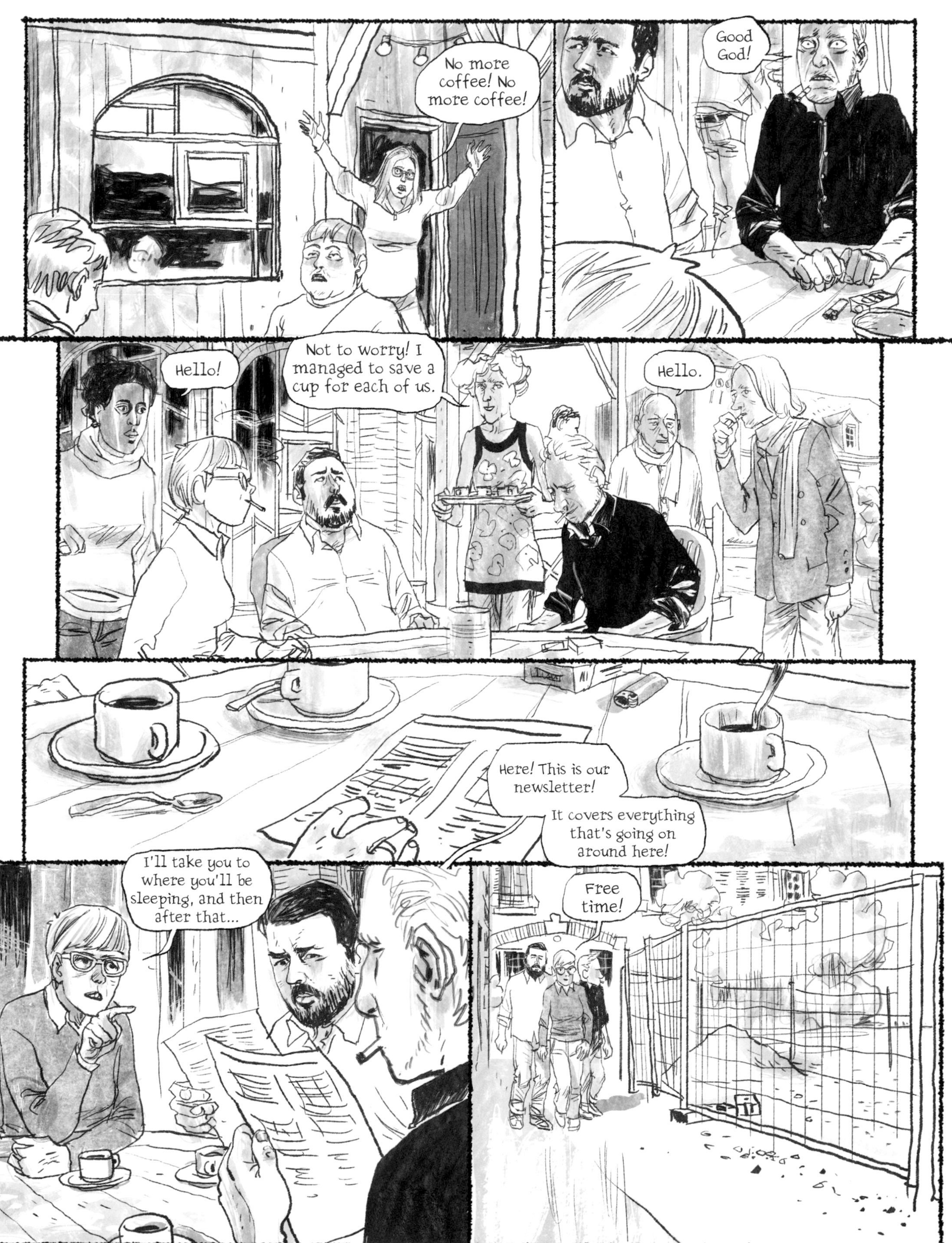
No more coffee! No more coffee!
Good God!
Hello!
Not to worry! I managed to save a cup for each of us.
Hello.
Here! This is our newsletter!
It covers everything that's going on around here!
I'll take you to where you'll be sleeping, and then after that...
Free time!

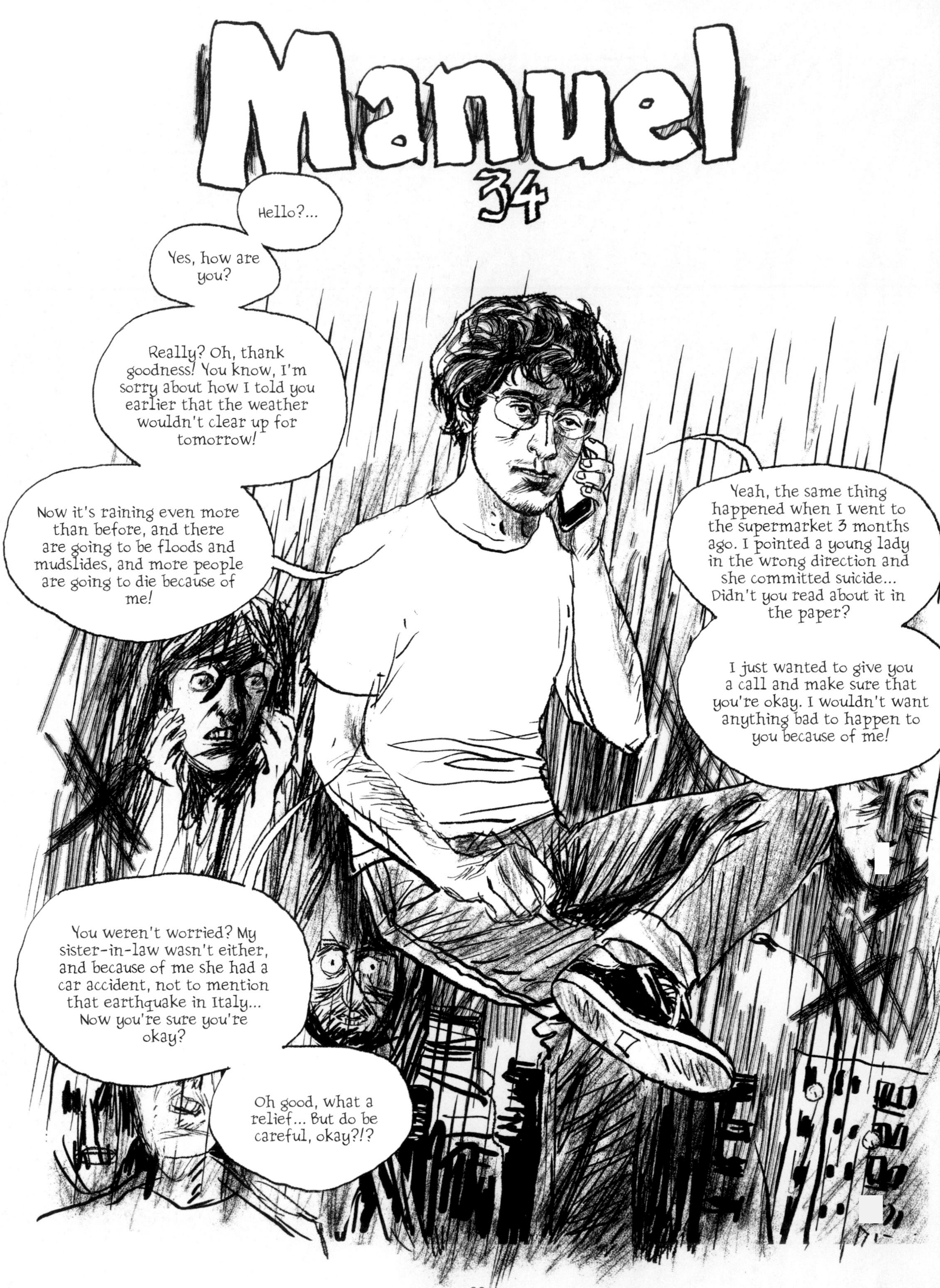
Manuel
34
Hello?...
Yes, how are you?
Really? Oh, thank goodness! You know, I'm sorry about how I told you earlier that the weather wouldn't clear up for tomorrow!
Now it's raining even more than before, and there are going to be floods and mudslides, and more people are going to die because of me!
Yeah, the same thing happened when I went to the supermarket 3 months ago. I pointed a young lady in the wrong direction and she committed suicide... Didn't you read about it in the paper?
I just wanted to give you a call and make sure that you're okay. I wouldn't want anything bad to happen to you because of me!
You weren't worried? My sister-in-law wasn't either, and because of me she had a car accident, not to mention that earthquake in Italy... Now you're sure you're okay?
Oh good, what a relief... But do be careful, okay?!?

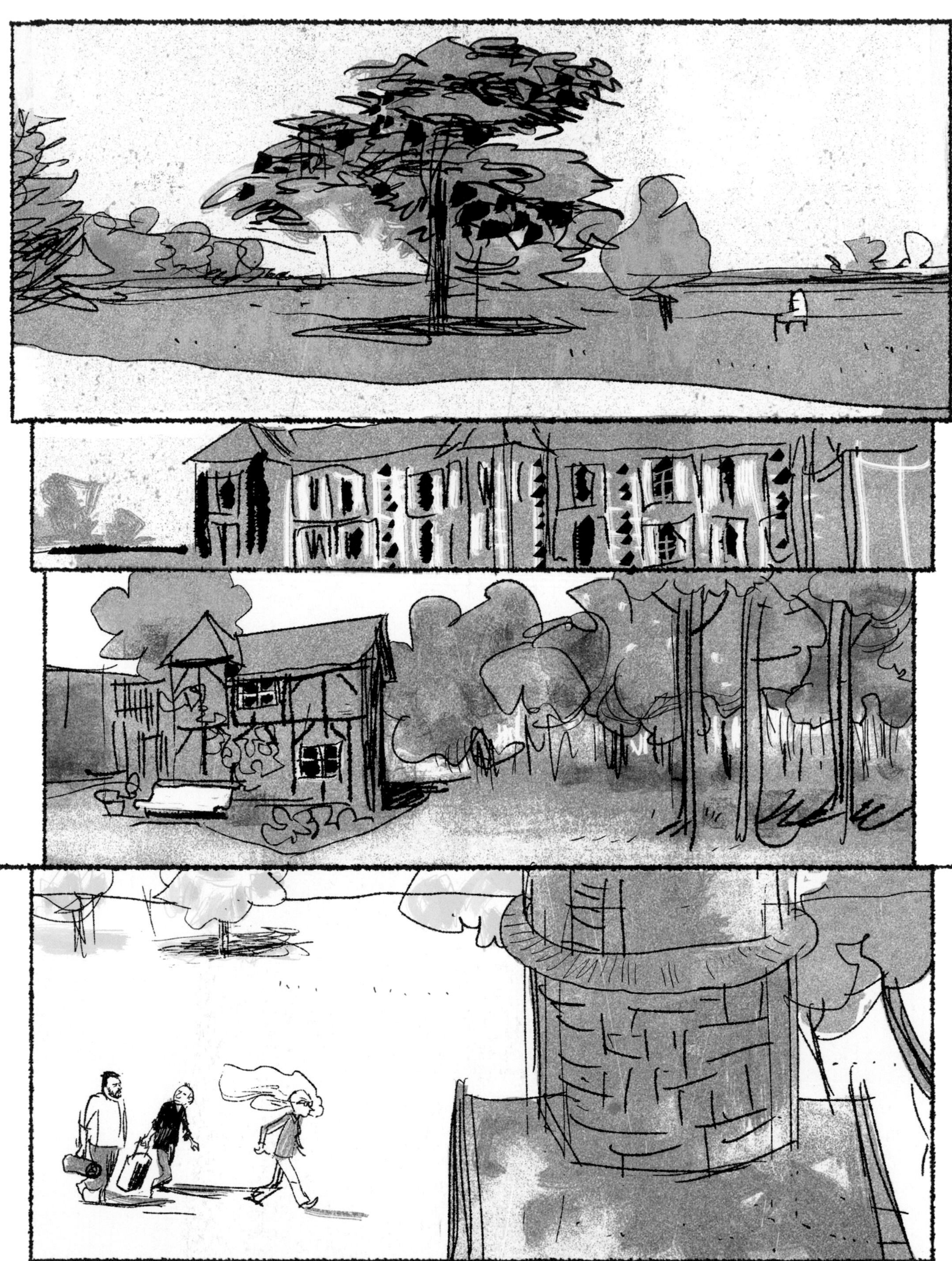

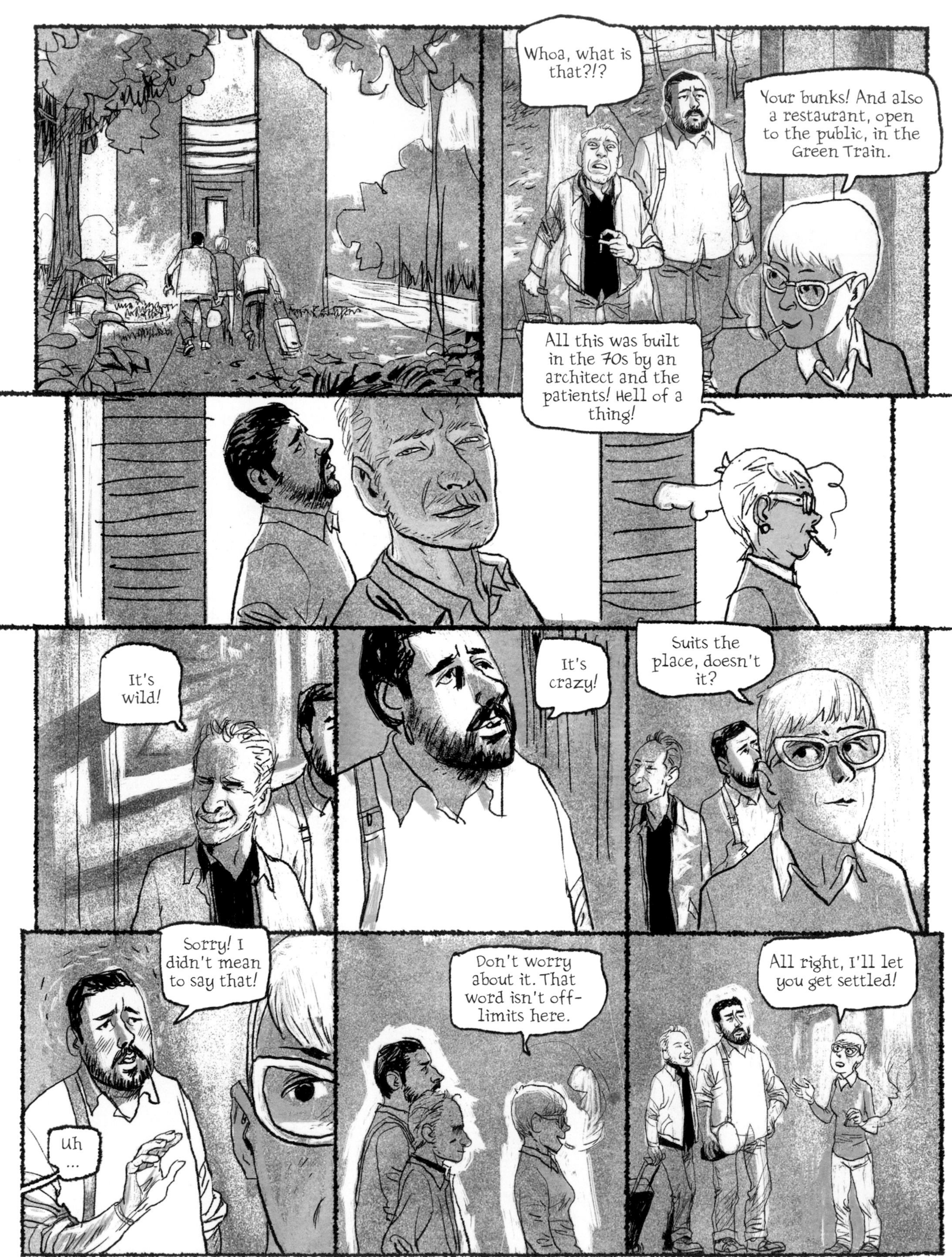
Whoa, what is that?!?
Your bunks! And also a restaurant, open to the public, in the Green Train.
All this was built in the 70s by an architect and the patients! Hell of a thing!
It's wild!
It's crazy!
Suits the place, doesn't it?
Sorry! I didn't mean to say that!
Uh ...
Don't worry about it. That word isn't off-limits here.
All right, I'll let you get settled!

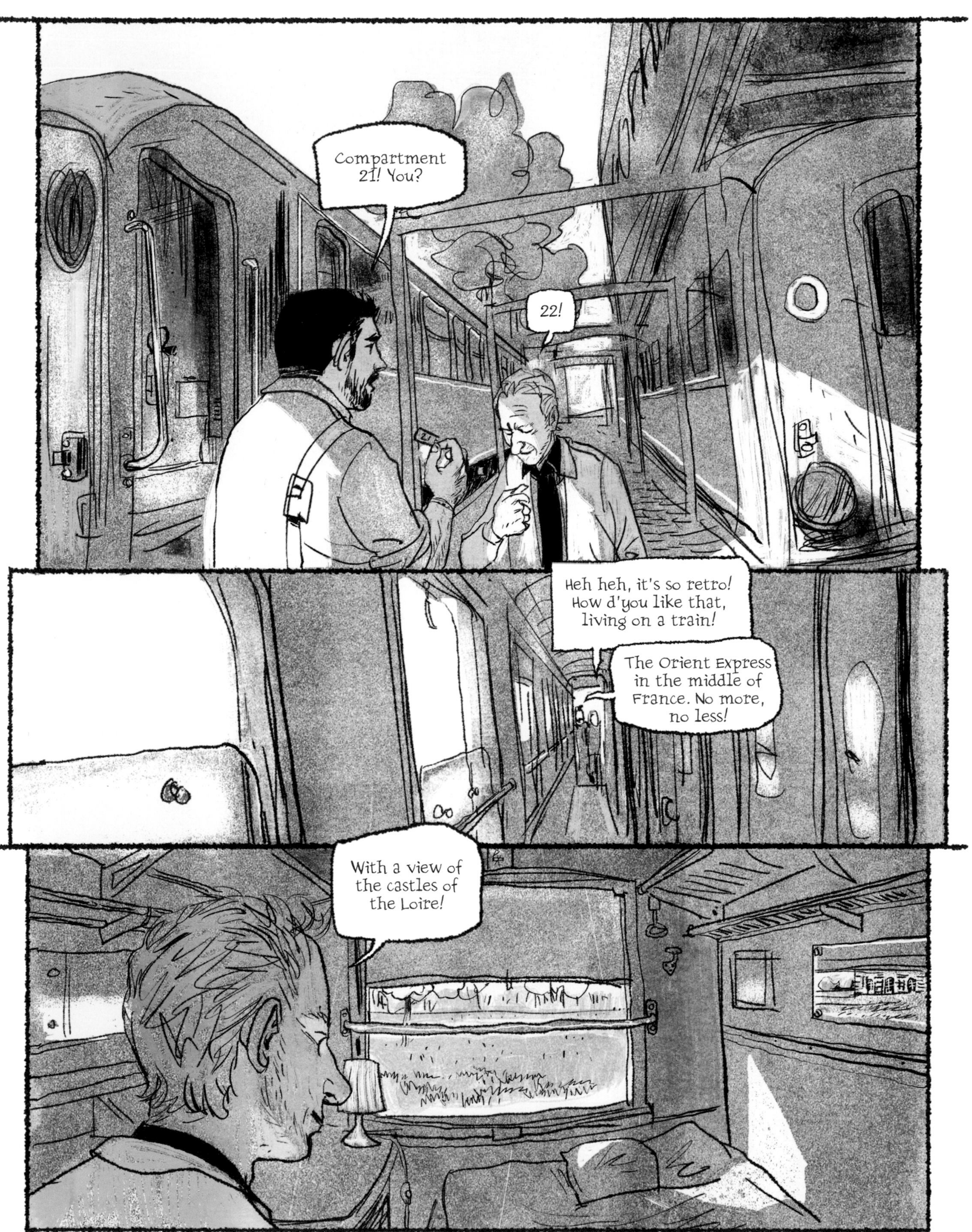
Compartment 21! You?
22!
Heh heh, it's so retro! How d'you like that, living on a train!
The Orient Express in the middle of France. No more, no less!
With a view of the castles of the Loire!

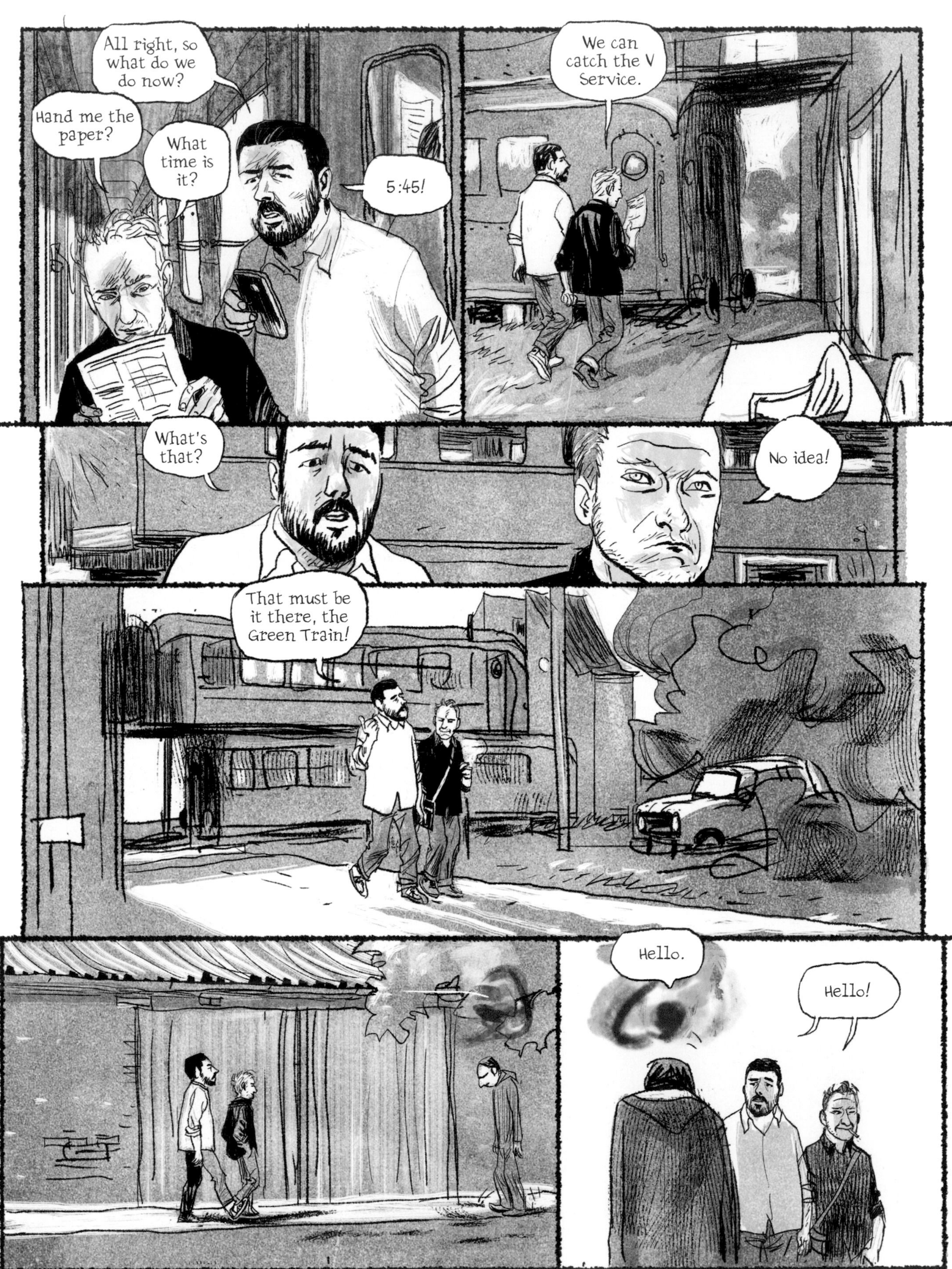
All right, so what do we do now?
Hand me the paper?
What time is it?
5:45!
We can catch the V Service.
What's that?
No idea!
That must be it there, the Green Train!
Hello.
Hello!

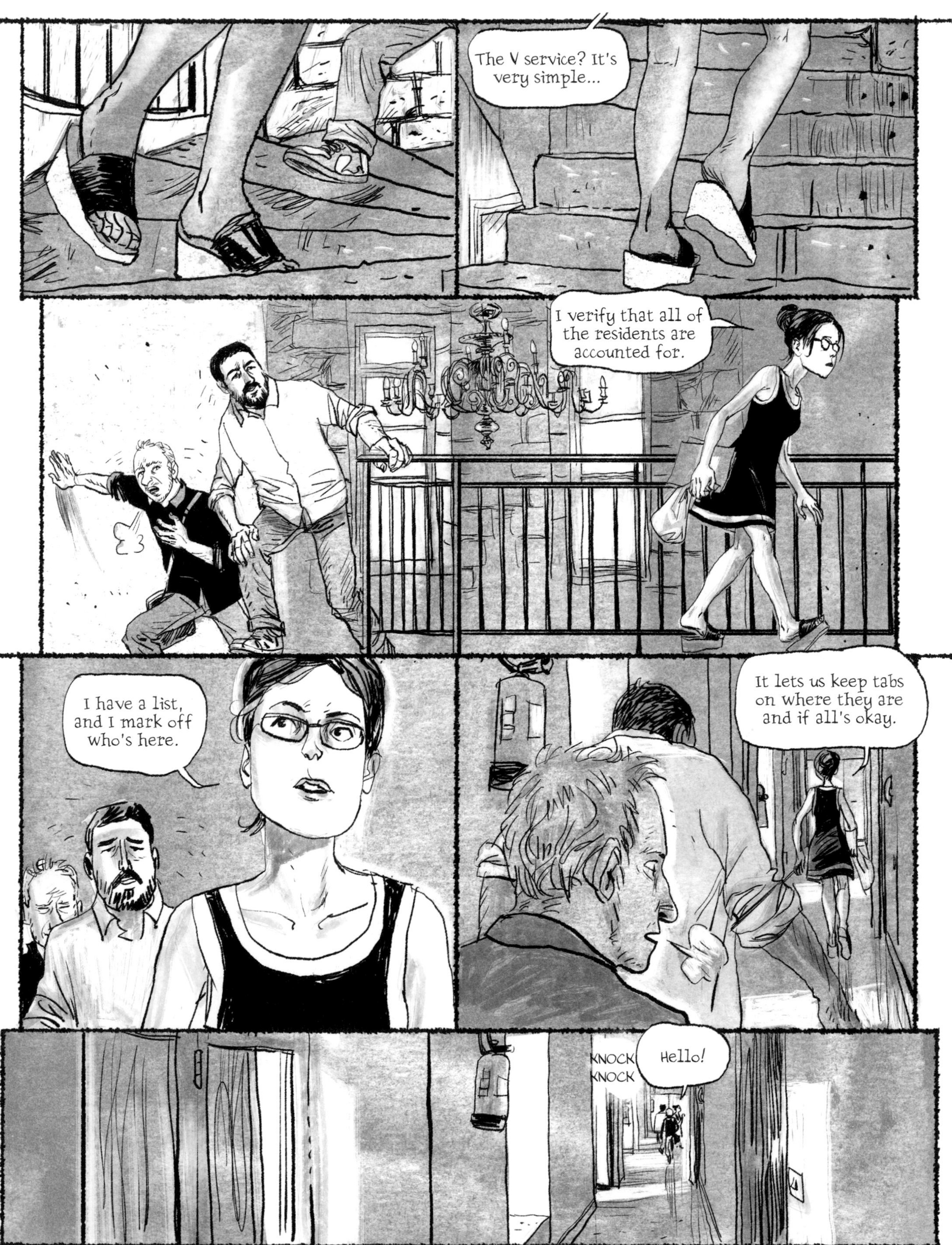
The V service? It's very simple...
I verify that all of the residents are accounted for.
I have a list, and I mark off who's here.
It lets us keep tabs on where they are and if all's okay.
KNOCK KNOCK
Hello!

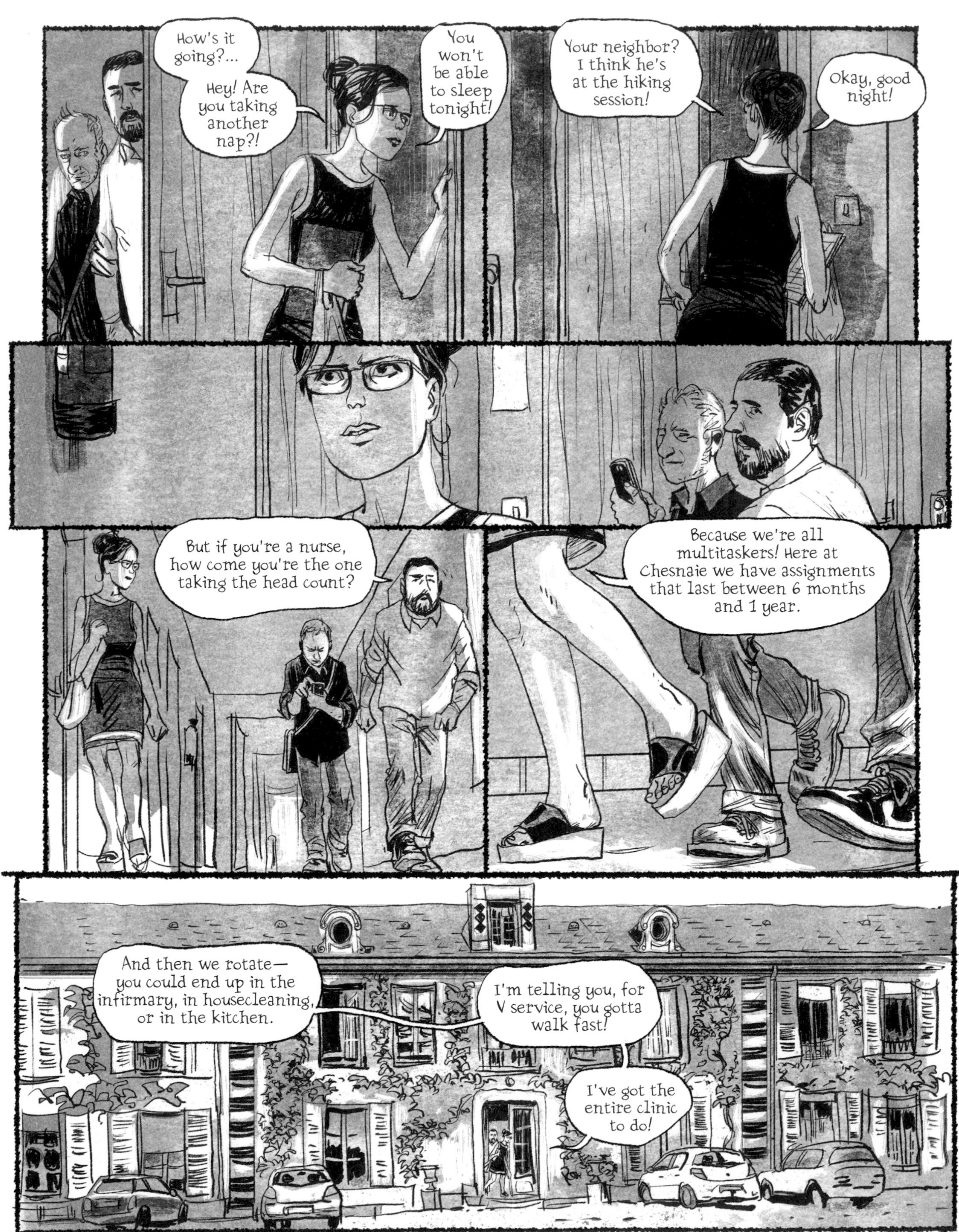
How's it going?...
Hey! Are you taking another nap?!
You won't be able to sleep tonight!
Your neighbor? I think he's at the hiking session!
Okay, good night!
But if you're a nurse, how come you're the one taking the head count?
Because we're all multitaskers! Here at Chesnaie we have assignments that last between 6 months and 1 year.
And then we rotate—you could end up in the infirmary, in housecleaning, or in the kitchen.
I'm telling you, for V service, you gotta walk fast!
I've got the entire clinic to do!

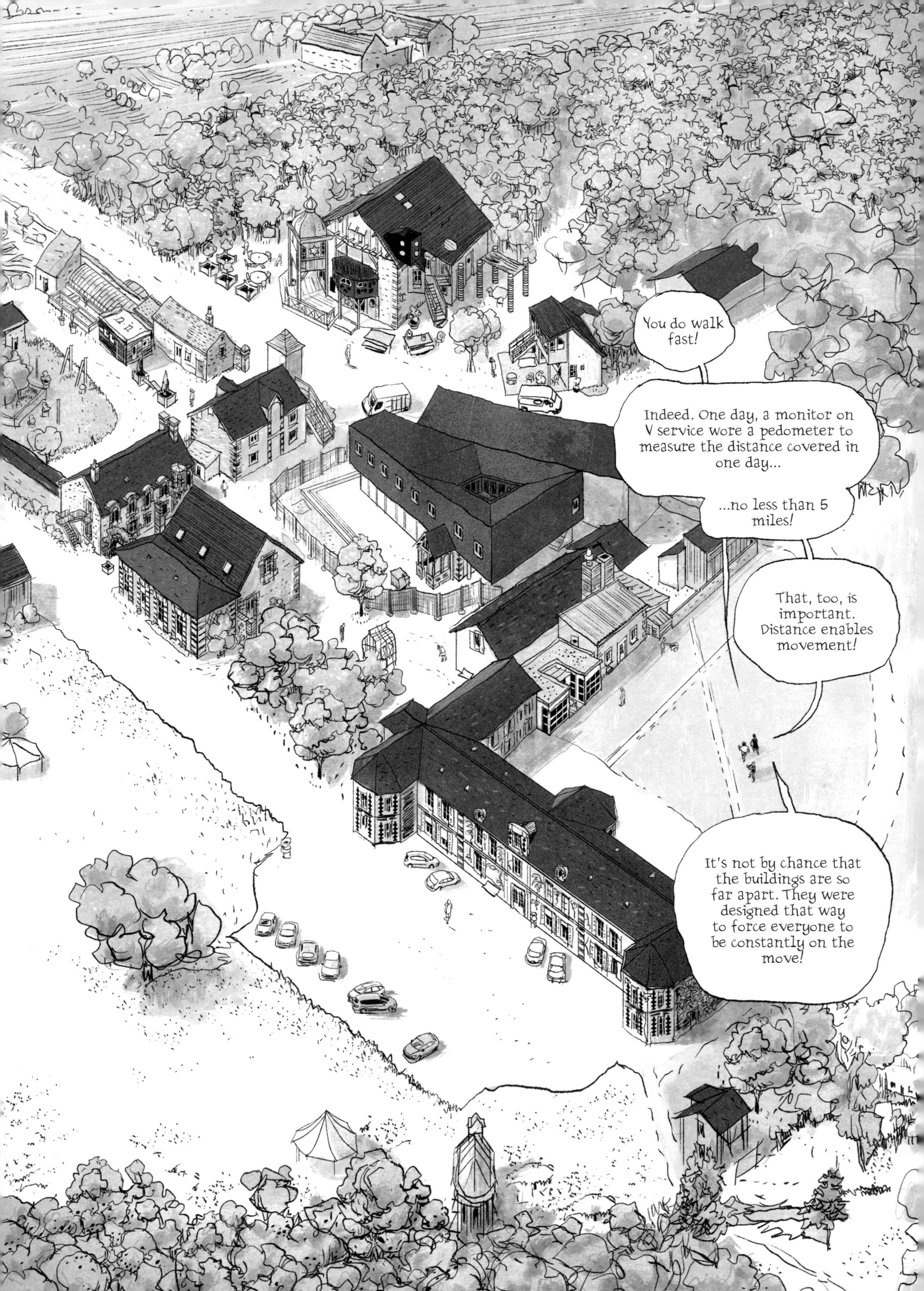
You do walk fast!
Indeed. One day, a monitor on V service wore a pedometer to measure the distance covered in one day...
...no less than 5 miles!
That, too, is important. Distance enables movement!
It's not by chance that the buildings are so far apart. They were designed that way to force everyone to be constantly on the move!

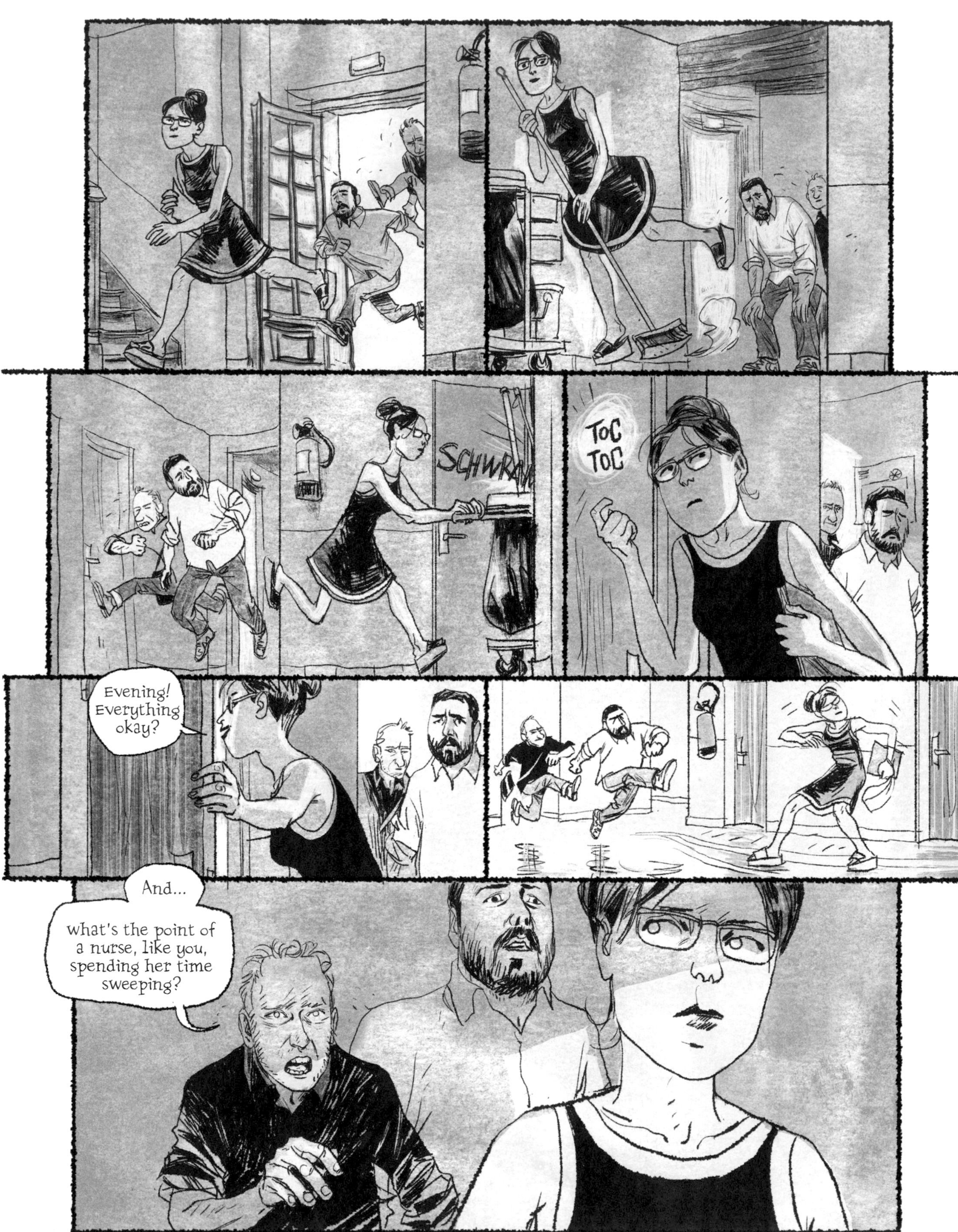
SCHWRAA
TOC TOC
Evening! Everything okay?
And...
what's the point of a nurse, like you, spending her time sweeping?

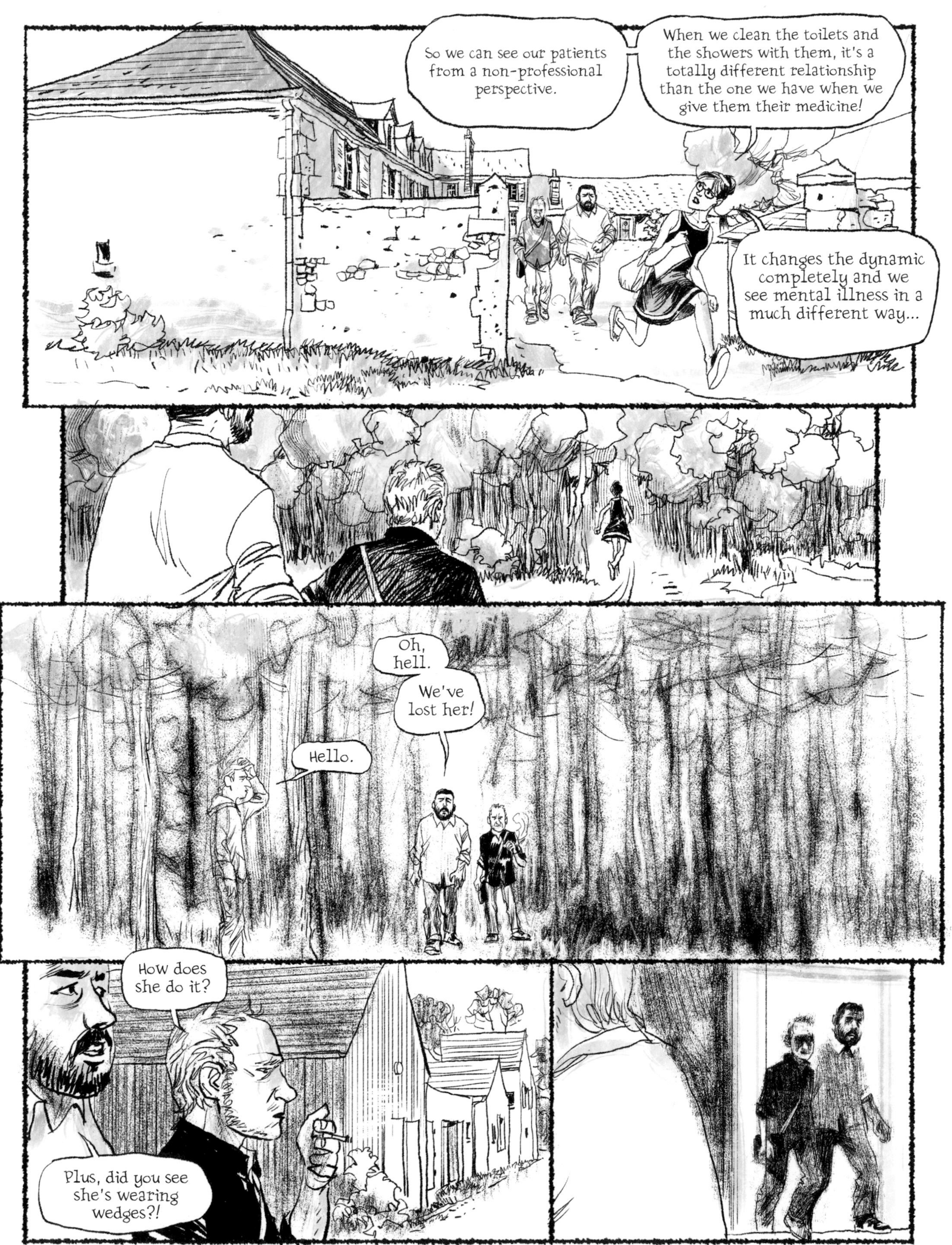
So we can see our patients from a non-professional perspective.
When we clean the toilets and the showers with them, it's a totally different relationship than the one we have when we give them their medicine!
It changes the dynamic completely and we see mental illness in a much different way...
Oh, hell.
We've lost her!
Hello.
How does she do it?
Plus, did you see she's wearing wedges?!

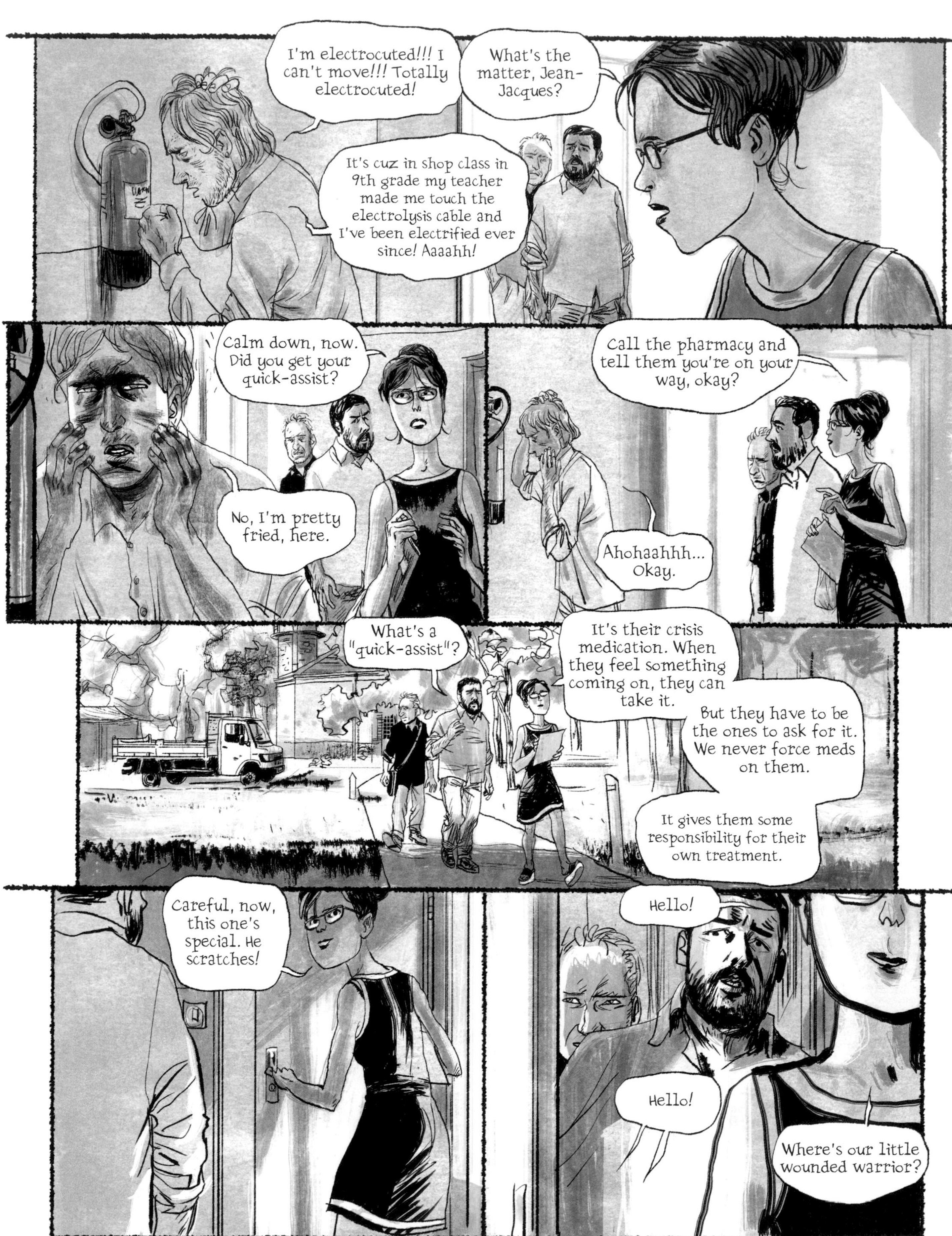
I'm electrocuted!!! I can't move!!! Totally electrocuted!
What's the matter, Jean-Jacques?
It's cuz in shop class in 9th grade my teacher made me touch the electrolysis cable and I've been electrified ever since! Aaaahh!
Calm down, now. Did you get your quick-assist?
No, I'm pretty fried, here.
Call the pharmacy and tell them you're on your way, okay?
Ahohaahhh... Okay.
What's a "quick-assist"?
It's their crisis medication. When they feel something coming on, they can take it.
But they have to be the ones to ask for it. We never force meds on them.
It gives them some responsibility for their own treatment.
Careful, now, this one's special. He scratches!
Hello!
Hello!
Where's our little wounded warrior?

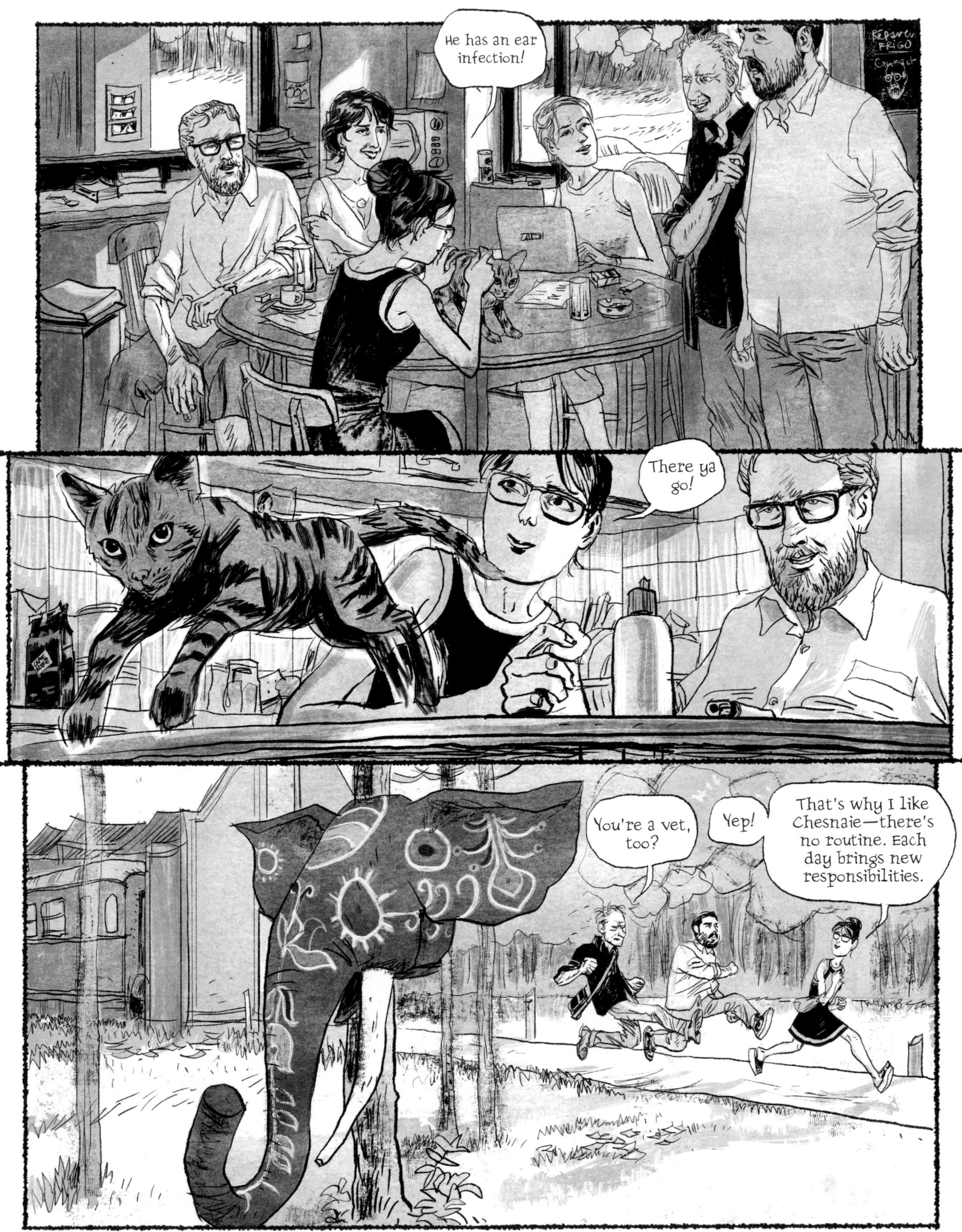
He has an ear infection!
There ya go!
You're a vet, too?
Yep!
That's why I like Chesnaie—there's no routine. Each day brings new responsibilities.

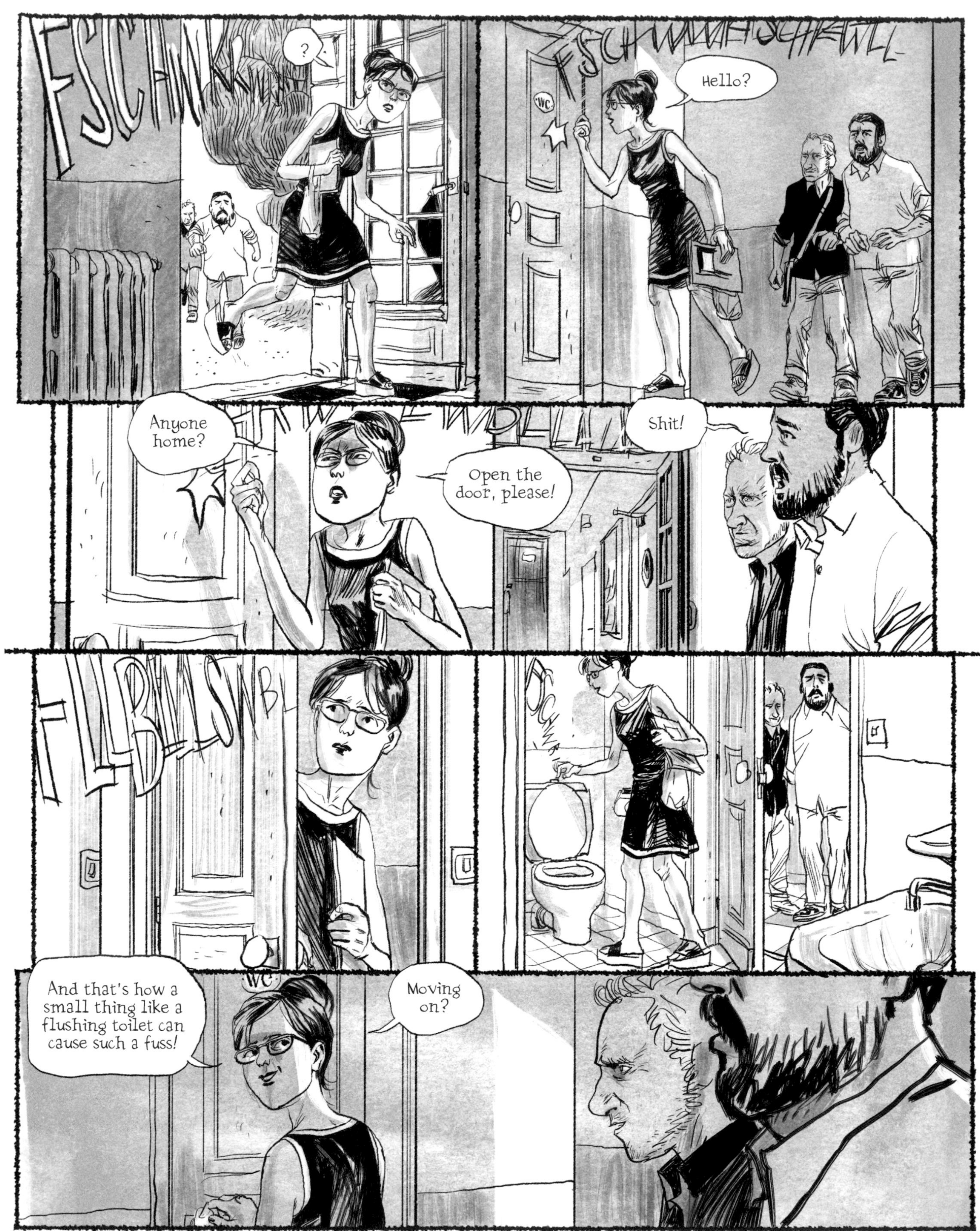
FSCHANK
?
FSCHWHSCHRWLL
Hello?
WC
Anyone home?
Open the door, please!
Shit!
And that's how a small thing like a flushing toilet can cause such a fuss!
Moving on?

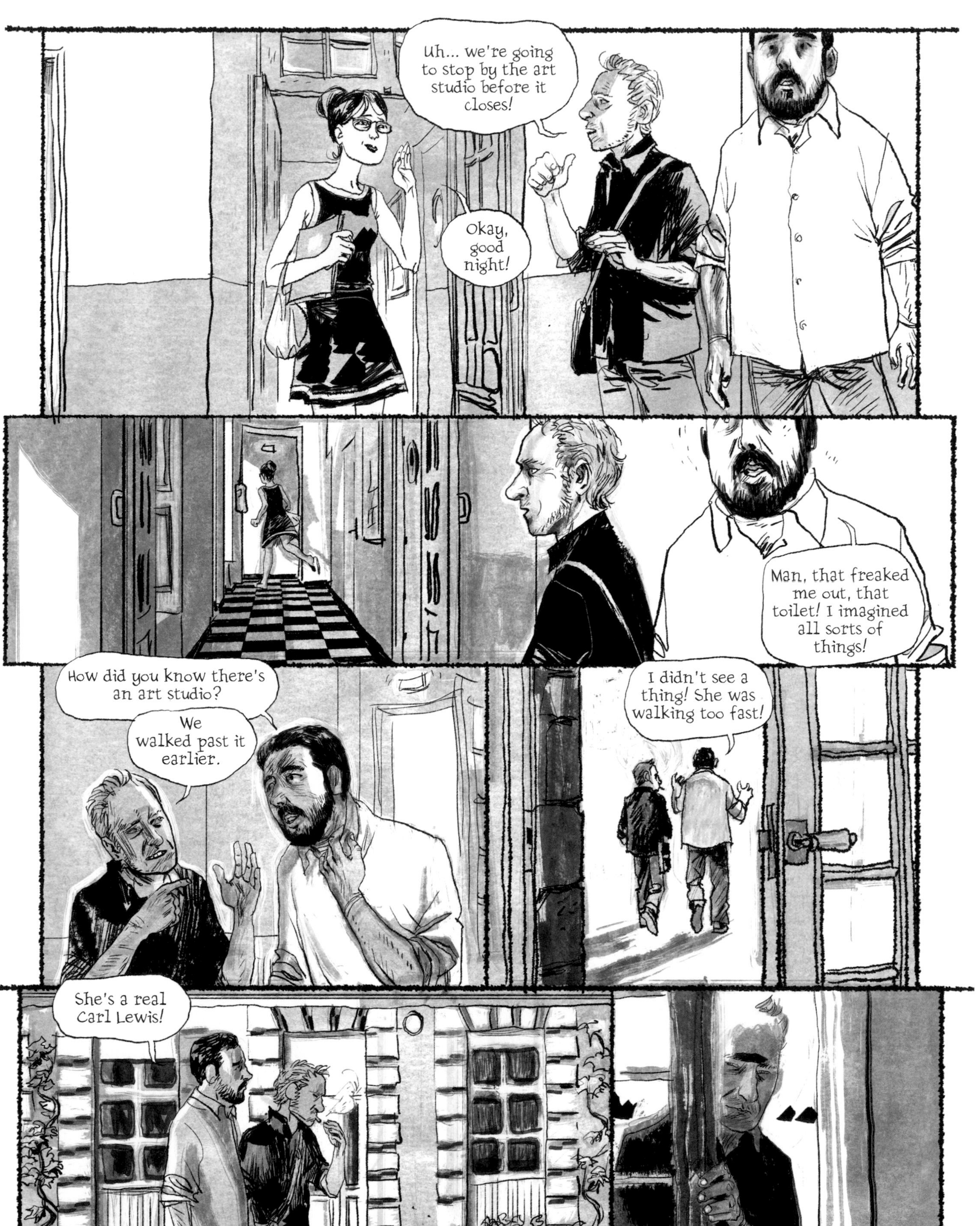
Uh... we're going to stop by the art studio before it closes!
Okay, good night!
Man, that freaked me out, that toilet! I imagined all sorts of things!
How did you know there's an art studio?
We walked past it earlier.
I didn't see a thing! She was walking too fast!
She's a real Carl Lewis!

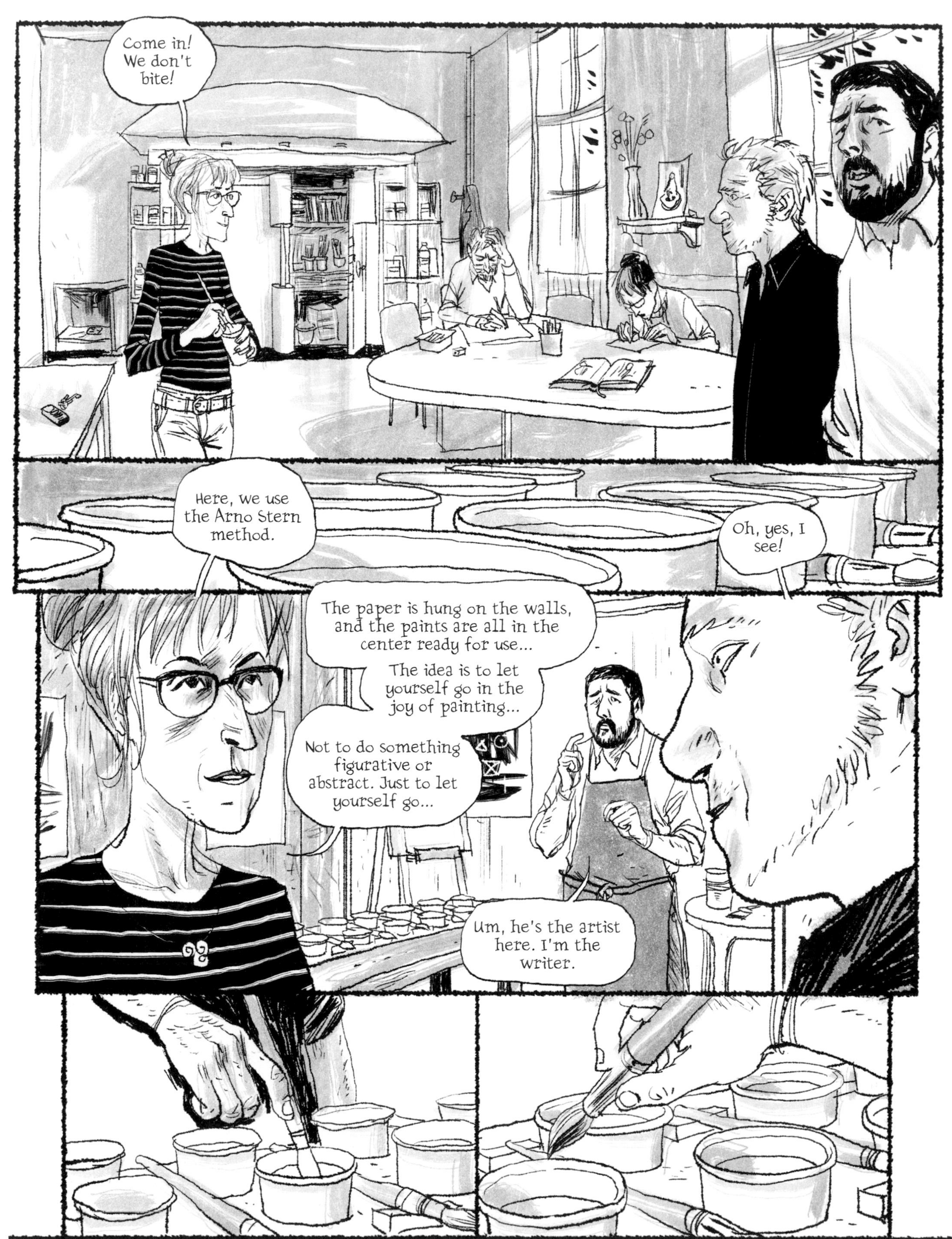

Come in! We don't bite!
Here, we use the Arno Stern method.
Oh, yes, I see!
The paper is hung on the walls, and the paints are all in the center ready for use...
The idea is to let yourself go in the joy of painting...
Not to do something figurative or abstract. Just to let yourself go...
Um, he's the artist here. I'm the writer.

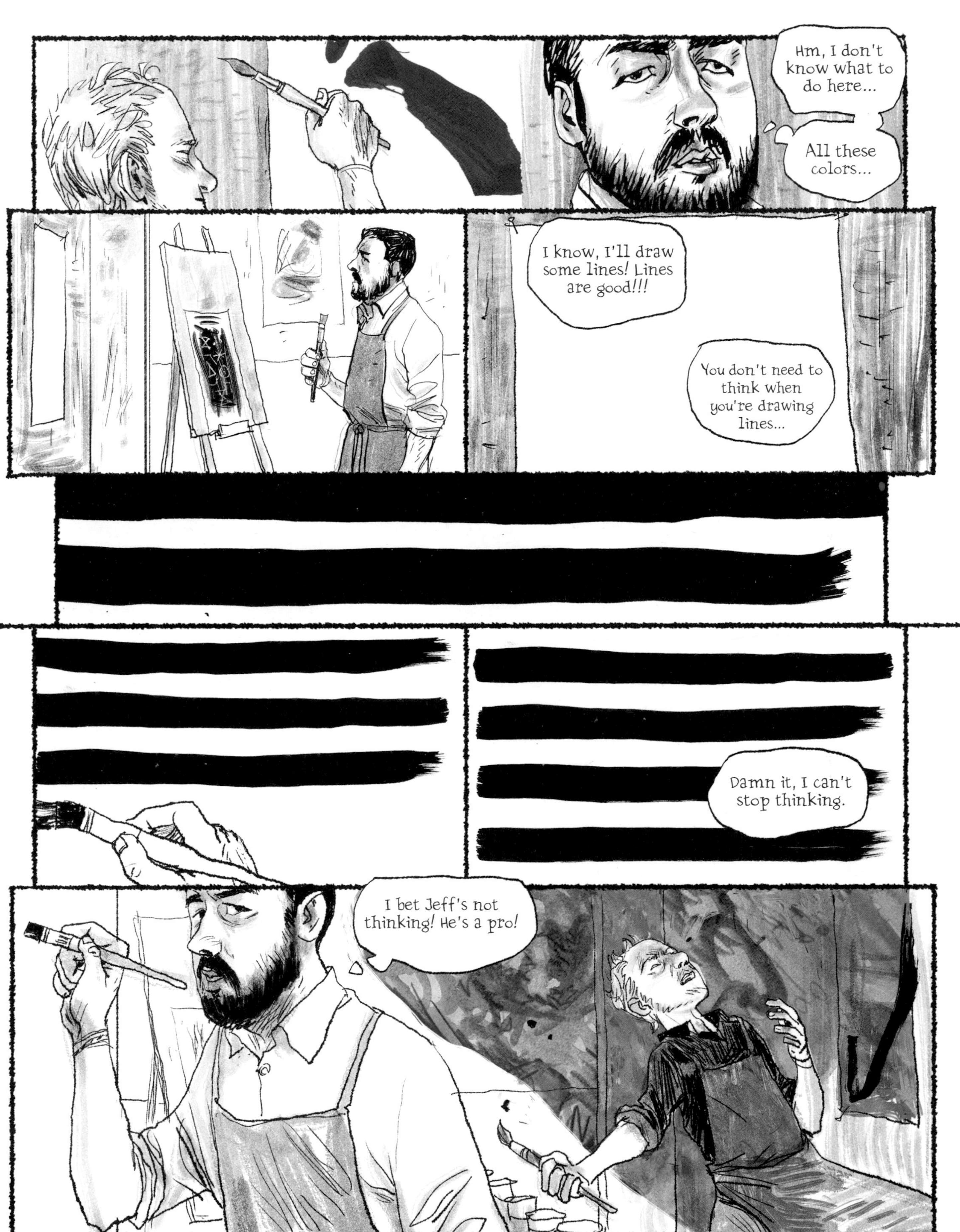
Hm, I don't know what to do here...
All these colors...
I know, I'll draw some lines! Lines are good!!!
You don't need to think when you're drawing lines...
Damn it, I can't stop thinking.
I bet Jeff's not thinking! He's a pro!

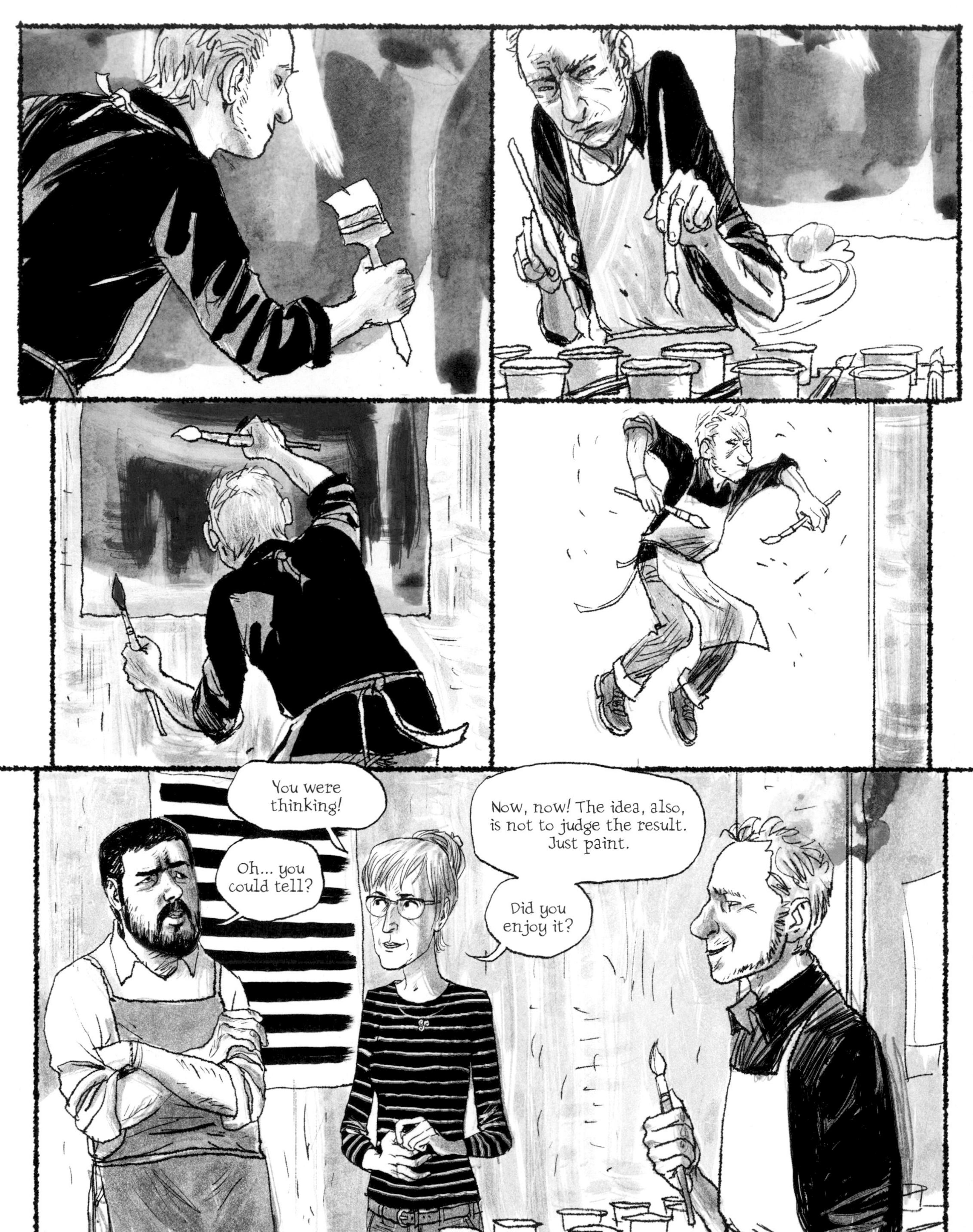
You were thinking!
Oh... you could tell?
Now, now! The idea, also, is not to judge the result. Just paint.
Did you enjoy it?

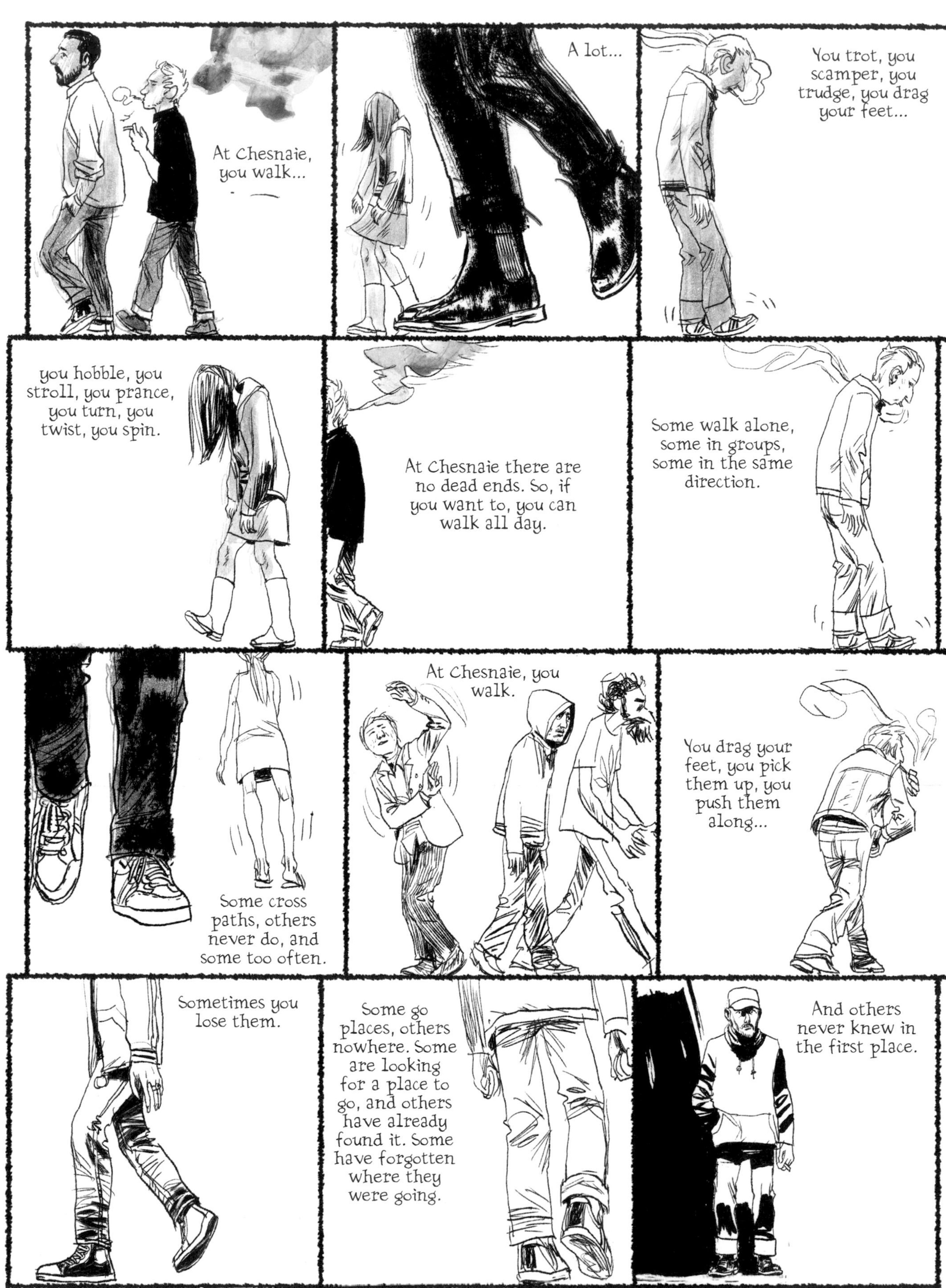
At Chesnaie,
you walk...
A lot...
You trot, you scamper, you trudge, you drag your feet...
you hobble, you stroll, you prance, you turn, you twist, you spin.
At Chesnaie there are no dead ends. So, if you want to, you can walk all day.
Some walk alone, some in groups, some in the same direction.
Some cross paths, others never do, and some too often.
At Chesnaie, you walk.
You drag your feet, you pick them up, you push them along...
Sometimes you lose them.
Some go places, others nowhere. Some are looking for a place to go, and others have already found it. Some have forgotten where they were going.
And others never knew in the first place.

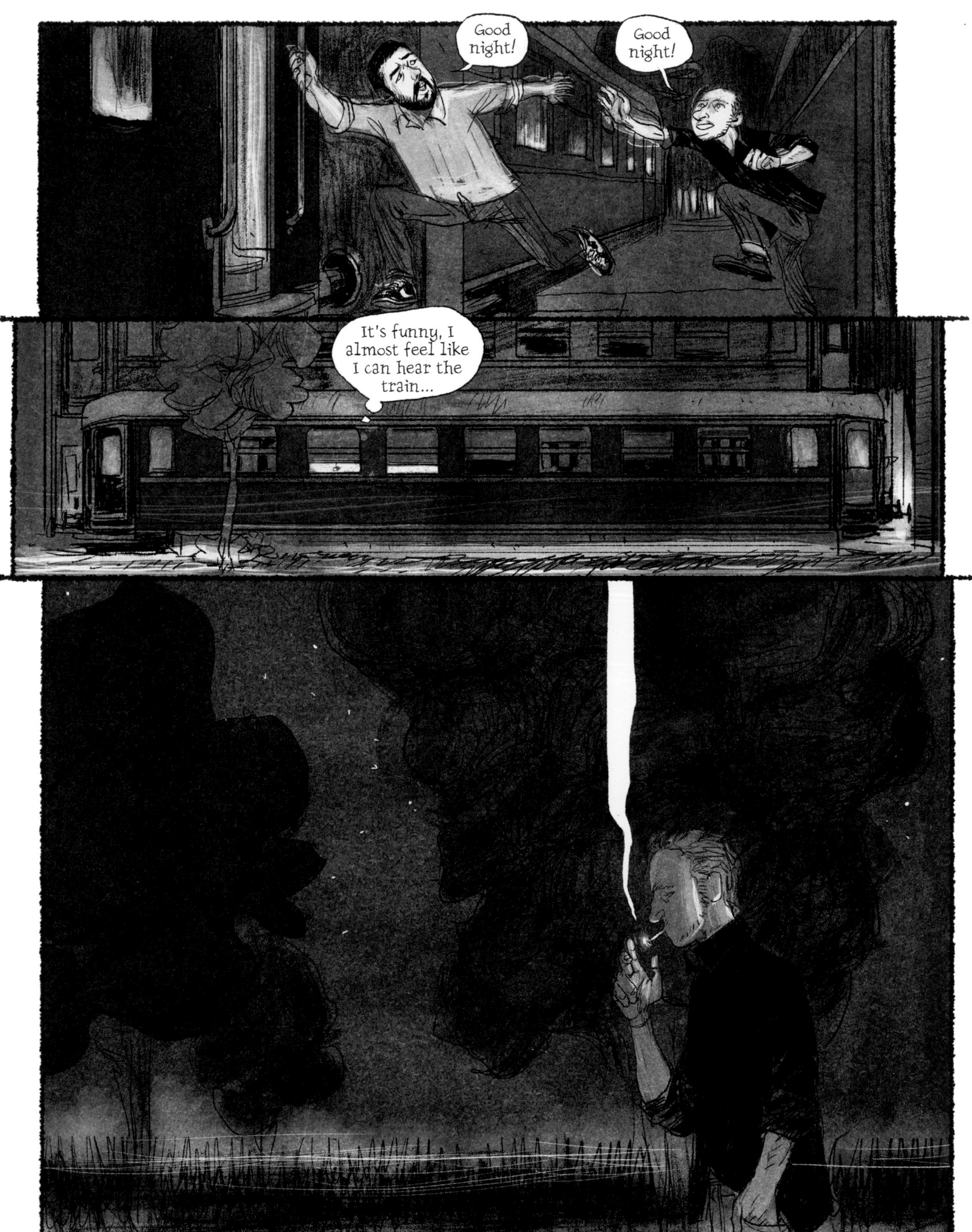
Good night!
Good night!
It's funny, I almost feel like I can hear the train...

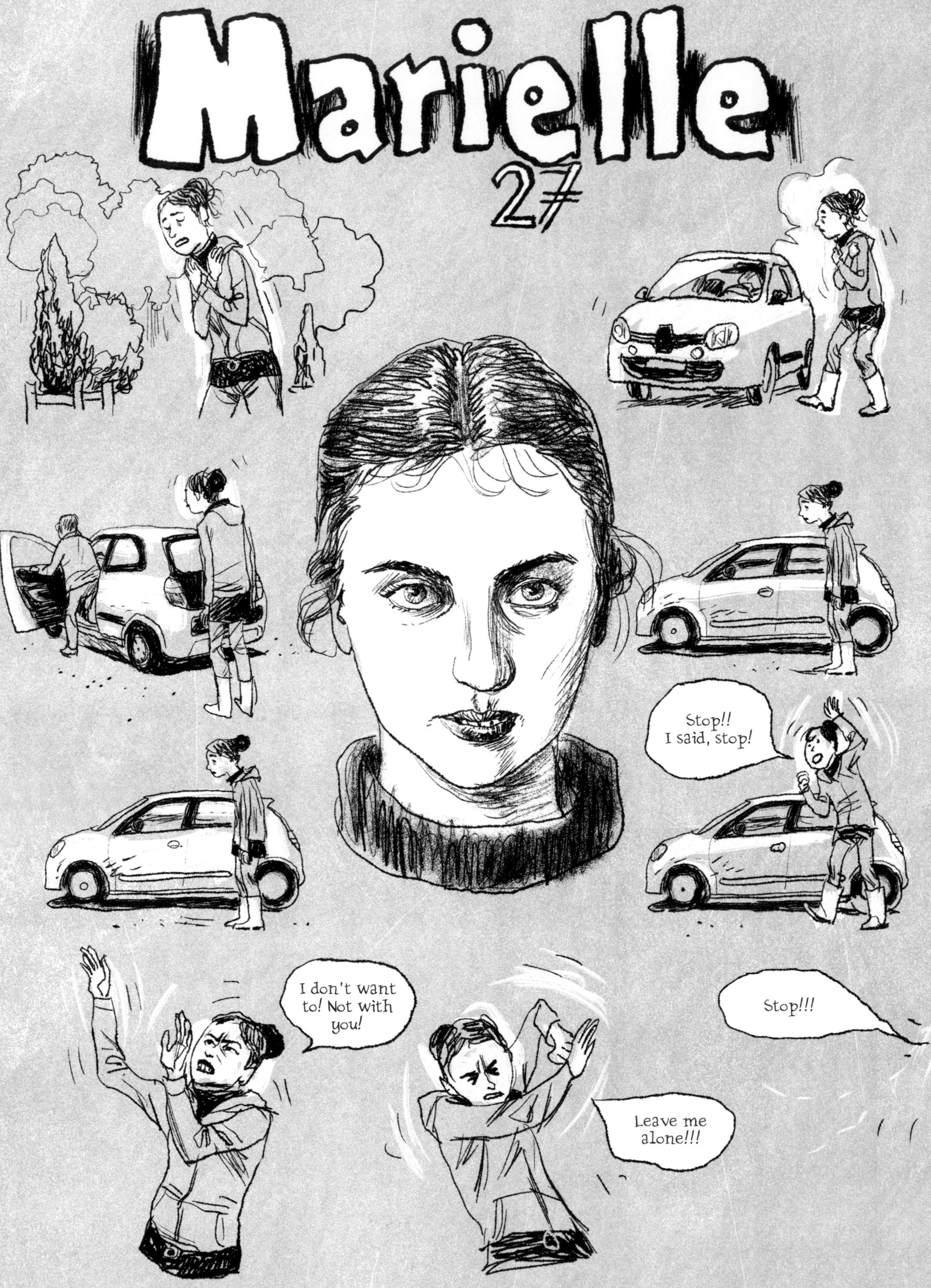

Marielle

27

Stop!!
I said, stop!

I don't want to! Not with you!

Stop!!!

Leave me alone!!!

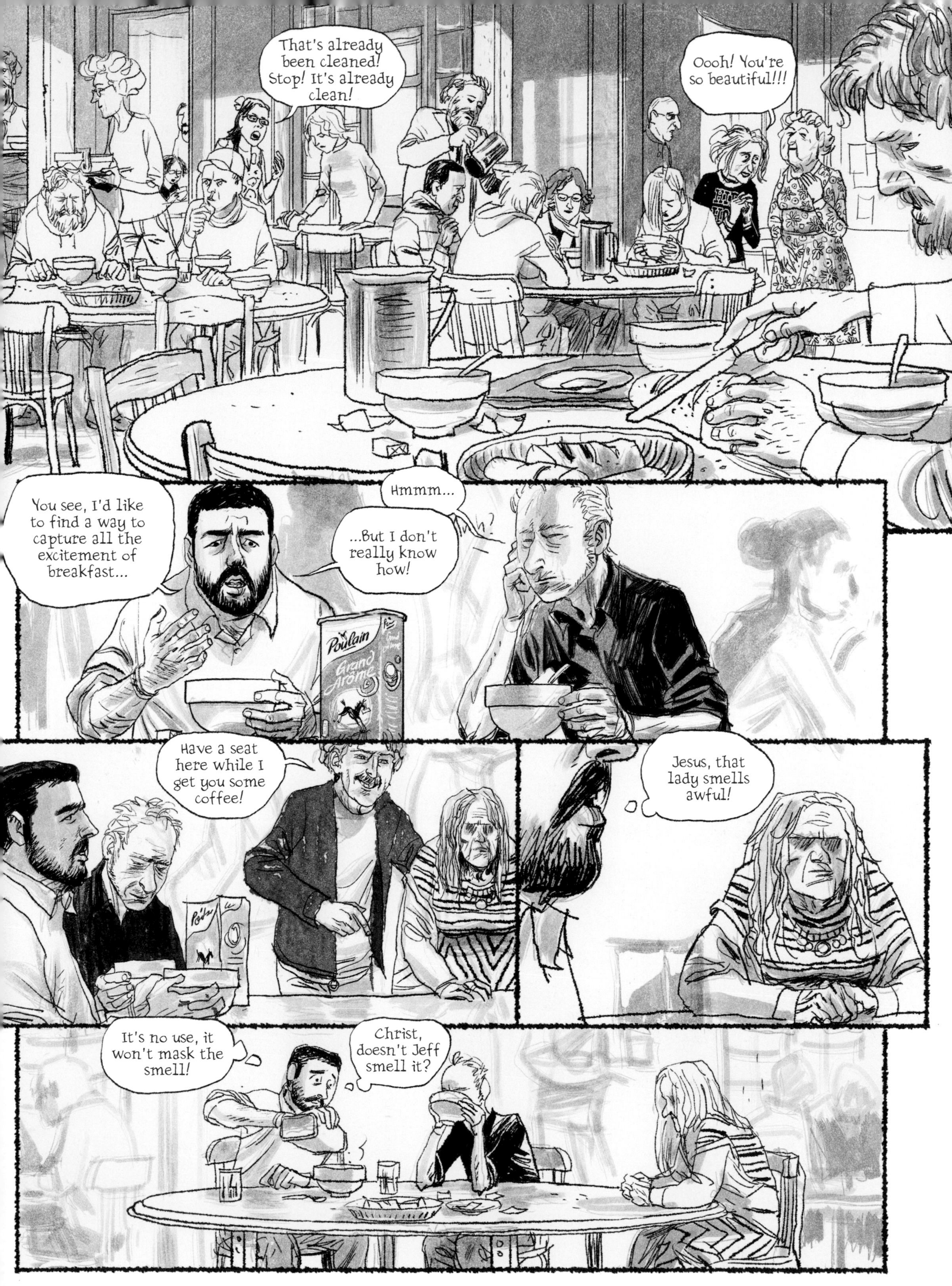

That's already been cleaned! Stop! It's already clean!
Oooh! You're so beautiful!!!
You see, I'd like to find a way to capture all the excitement of breakfast...
Hmmm...
...But I don't really know how!
Poulain
Grand Arôme
Have a seat here while I get you some coffee!
Jesus, that lady smells awful!
It's no use, it won't mask the smell!
Christ, doesn't Jeff smell it?

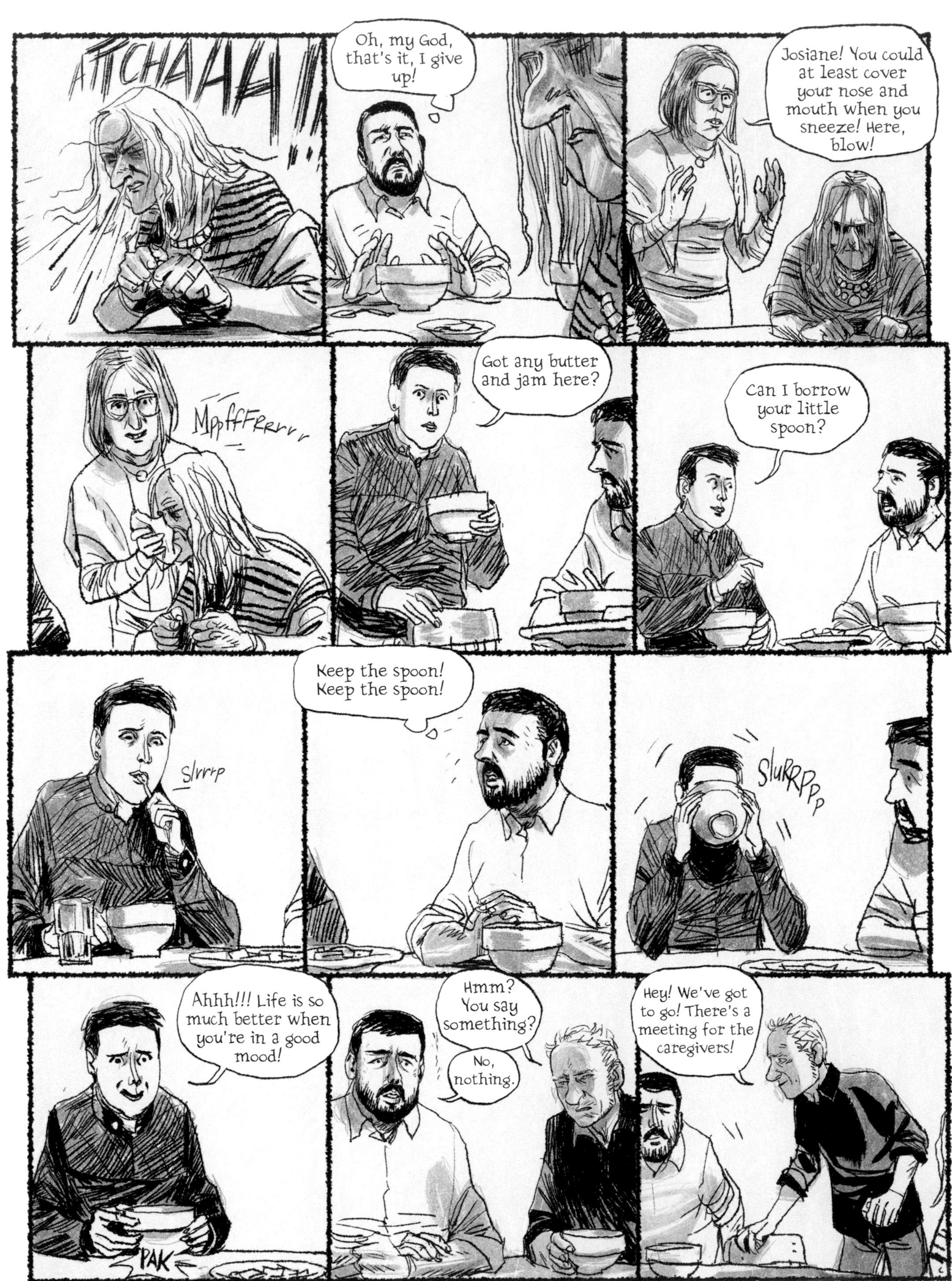
ATCHAAH!!
Oh, my God, that's it, I give up!
Josiane! You could at least cover your nose and mouth when you sneeze! Here, blow!
MPPFFFRRRRR
Got any butter and jam here?
Can I borrow your little spoon?
Slrrrp
Keep the spoon! Keep the spoon!
SLURRPPP
Ahhh!!! Life is so much better when you're in a good mood!
PAK
Hmm? You say something?
No, nothing.
Hey! We've got to go! There's a meeting for the caregivers!

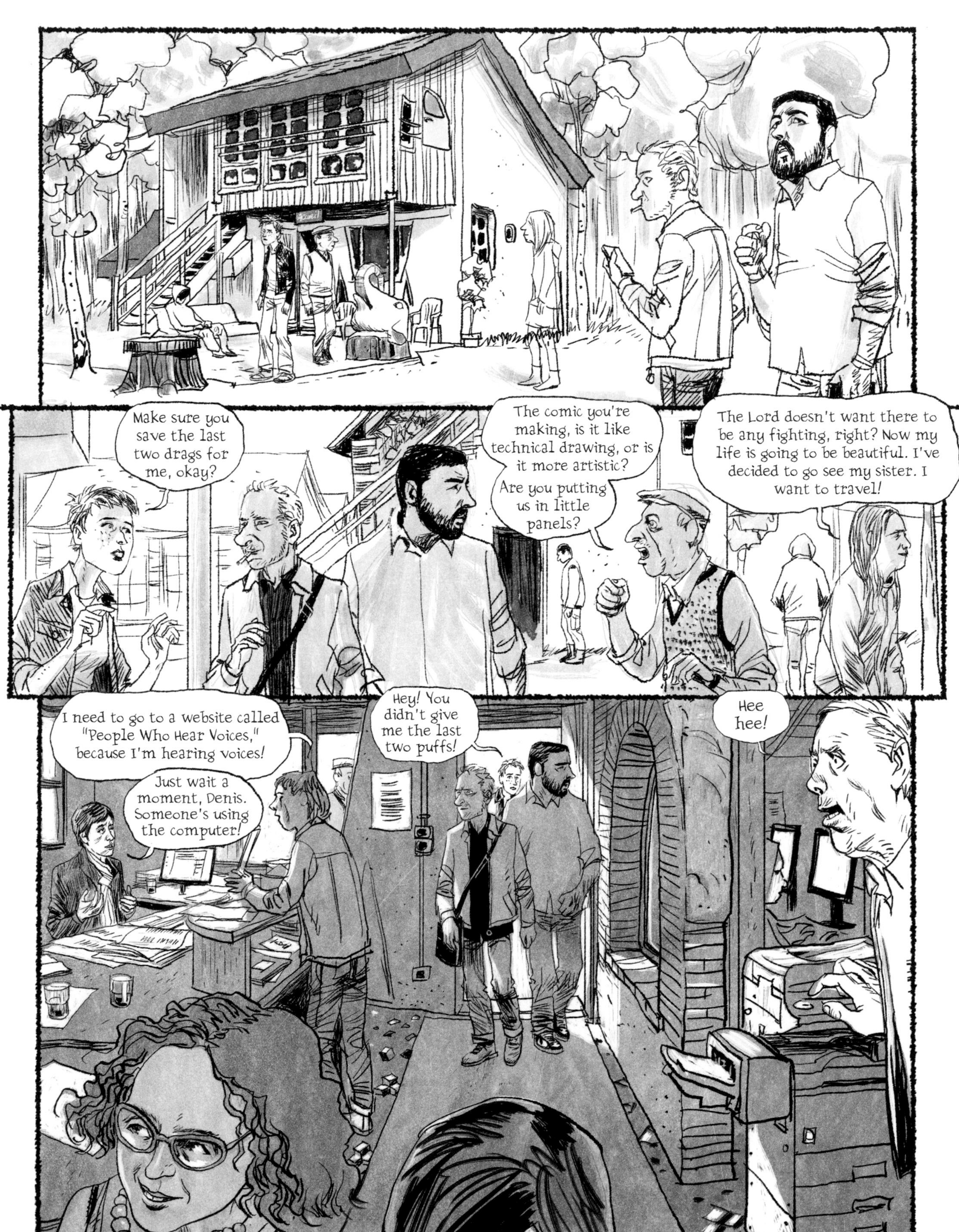
Make sure you save the last two drags for me, okay?
The comic you're making, is it like technical drawing, or is it more artistic?
Are you putting us in little panels?
The Lord doesn't want there to be any fighting, right? Now my life is going to be beautiful. I've decided to go see my sister. I want to travel!
I need to go to a website called "People Who Hear Voices," because I'm hearing voices!
Just wait a moment, Denis. Someone's using the computer!
Hey! You didn't give me the last two puffs!
Hee hee!

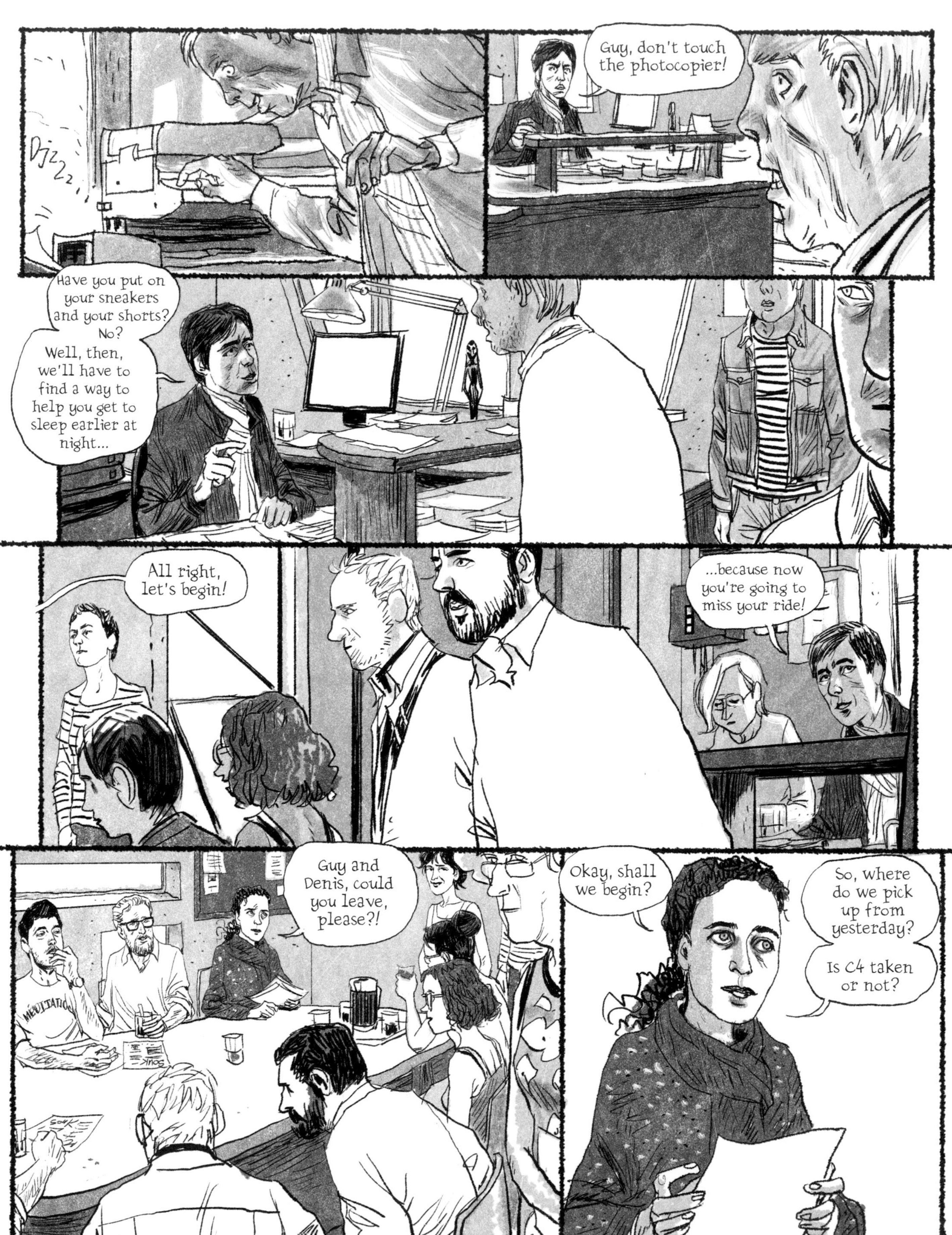
Djz z z
Guy, don't touch the photocopier!
Have you put on your sneakers and your shorts? No?
Well, then, we'll have to find a way to help you get to sleep earlier at night...
All right, let's begin!
...because now you're going to miss your ride!
Guy and Denis, could you leave, please?!
Okay, shall we begin?
So, where do we pick up from yesterday?
Is C4 taken or not?

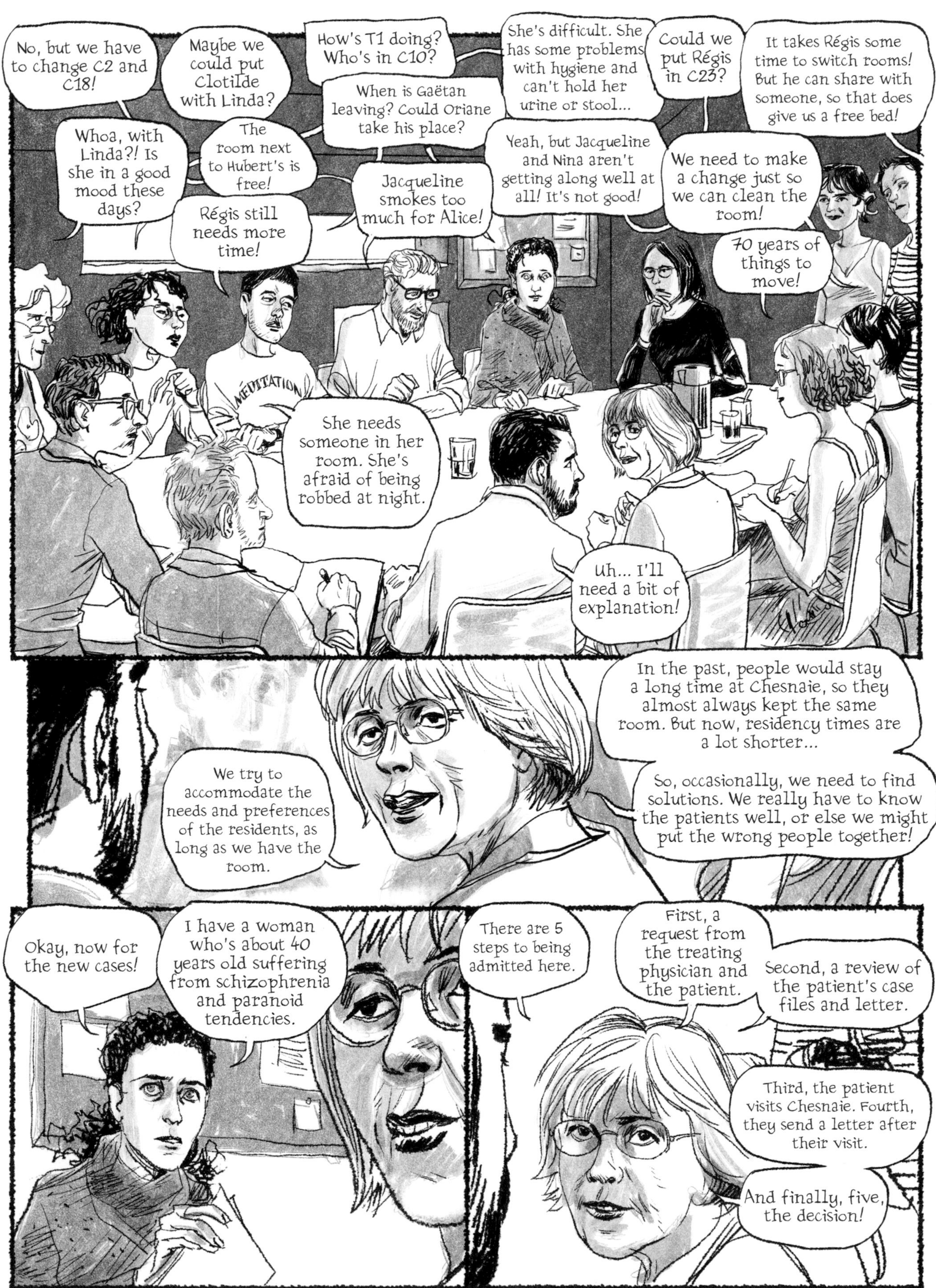
No, but we have to change C2 and C18!
Maybe we could put Clotilde with Linda?
How's T1 doing? Who's in C10?
She's difficult. She has some problems with hygiene and can't hold her urine or stool...
Could we put Régis in C23?
It takes Régis some time to switch rooms! But he can share with someone, so that does give us a free bed!
Whoa, with Linda?! Is she in a good mood these days?
The room next to Hubert's is free!
When is Gaëtan leaving? Could Oriane take his place?
Yeah, but Jacqueline and Nina aren't getting along well at all! It's not good!
We need to make a change just so we can clean the room!
Régis still needs more time!
Jacqueline smokes too much for Alice!
70 years of things to move!
MEDITATION
She needs someone in her room. She's afraid of being robbed at night.
Uh... I'll need a bit of explanation!
In the past, people would stay a long time at Chesnaie, so they almost always kept the same room. But now, residency times are a lot shorter...
We try to accommodate the needs and preferences of the residents, as long as we have the room.
So, occasionally, we need to find solutions. We really have to know the patients well, or else we might put the wrong people together!
Okay, now for the new cases!
I have a woman who's about 40 years old suffering from schizophrenia and paranoid tendencies.
There are 5 steps to being admitted here.
First, a request from the treating physician and the patient.
Second, a review of the patient's case files and letter.
Third, the patient visits Chesnaie. Fourth, they send a letter after their visit.
And finally, five, the decision!

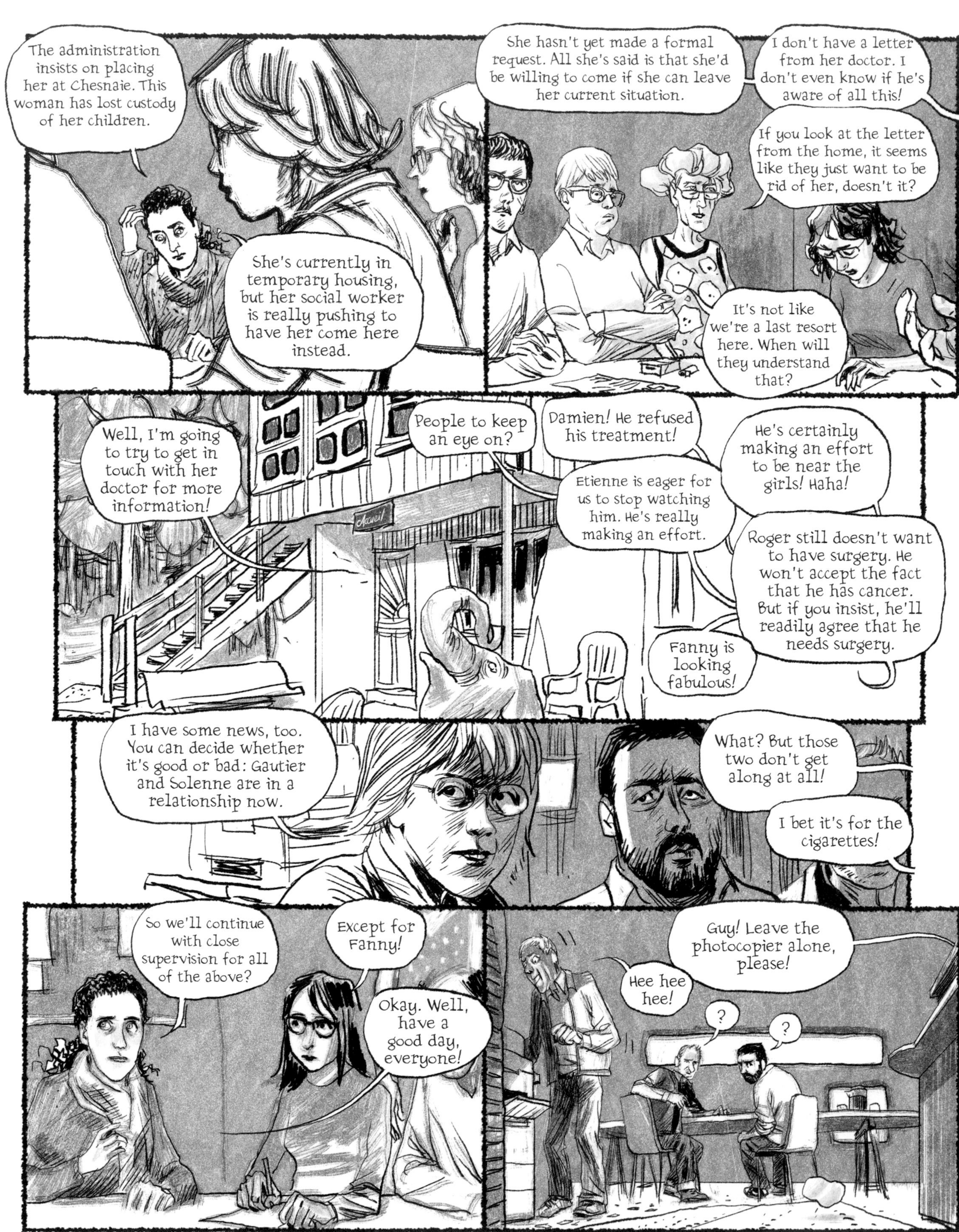
The administration insists on placing her at Chesnaie. This woman has lost custody of her children.
She's currently in temporary housing, but her social worker is really pushing to have her come here instead.
She hasn't yet made a formal request. All she's said is that she'd be willing to come if she can leave her current situation.
I don't have a letter from her doctor. I don't even know if he's aware of all this!
If you look at the letter from the home, it seems like they just want to be rid of her, doesn't it?
It's not like we're a last resort here. When will they understand that?
Well, I'm going to try to get in touch with her doctor for more information!
Accueil
People to keep an eye on?
Damien! He refused his treatment!
Etienne is eager for us to stop watching him. He's really making an effort.
He's certainly making an effort to be near the girls! Haha!
Roger still doesn't want to have surgery. He won't accept the fact that he has cancer. But if you insist, he'll readily agree that he needs surgery.
Fanny is looking fabulous!
I have some news, too. You can decide whether it's good or bad: Gautier and Solenne are in a relationship now.
What? But those two don't get along at all!
I bet it's for the cigarettes!
So we'll continue with close supervision for all of the above?
Except for Fanny!
Okay. Well, have a good day, everyone!
Guy! Leave the photocopier alone, please!
Hee hee hee!
?
?

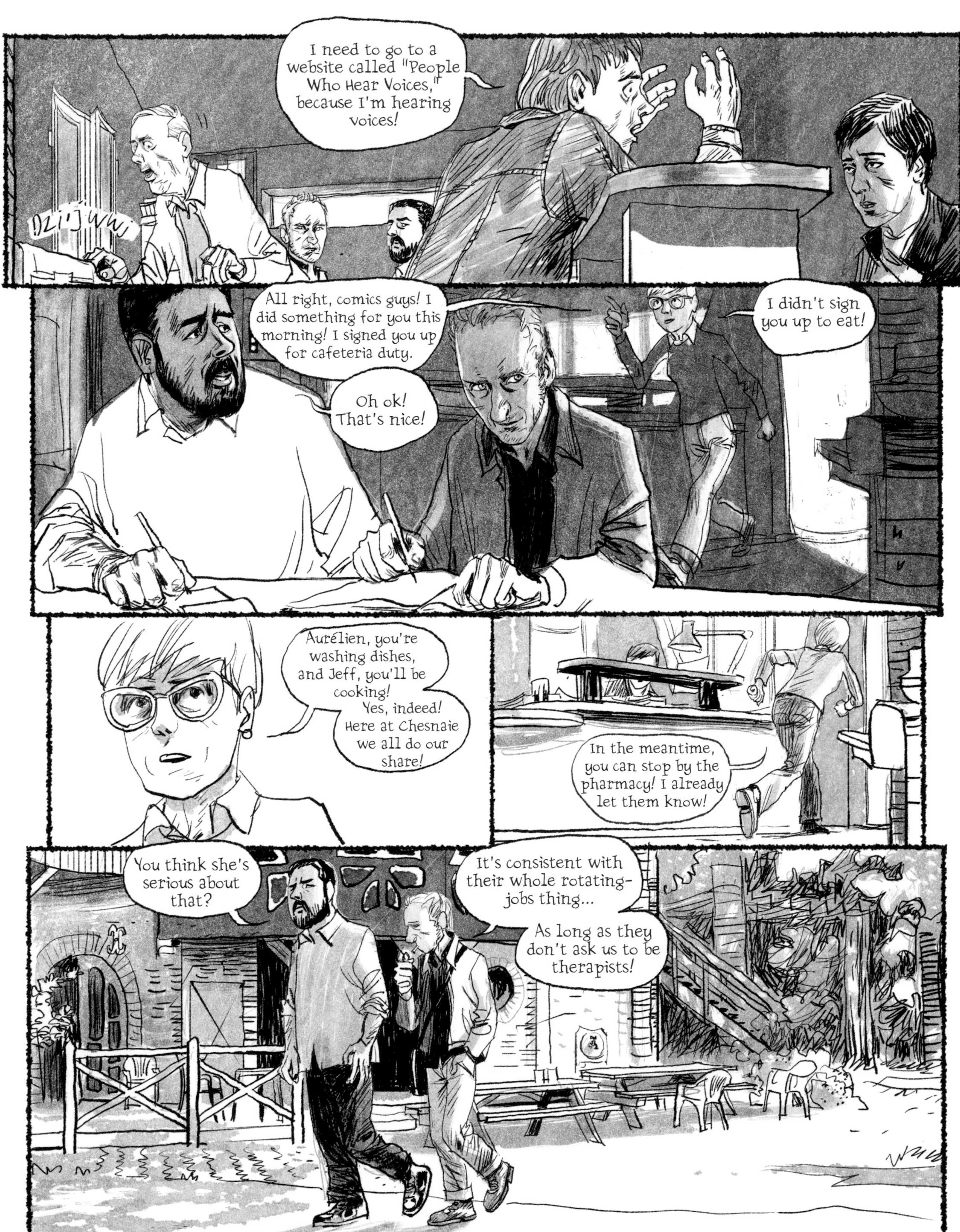
I need to go to a website called "People Who Hear Voices," because I'm hearing voices!
All right, comics guys! I did something for you this morning! I signed you up for cafeteria duty.
Oh ok! That's nice!
I didn't sign you up to eat!
Aurélien, you're washing dishes, and Jeff, you'll be cooking!
Yes, indeed! Here at Chesnaie we all do our share!
In the meantime, you can stop by the pharmacy! I already let them know!
You think she's serious about that?
It's consistent with their whole rotating-jobs thing...
As long as they don't ask us to be therapists!

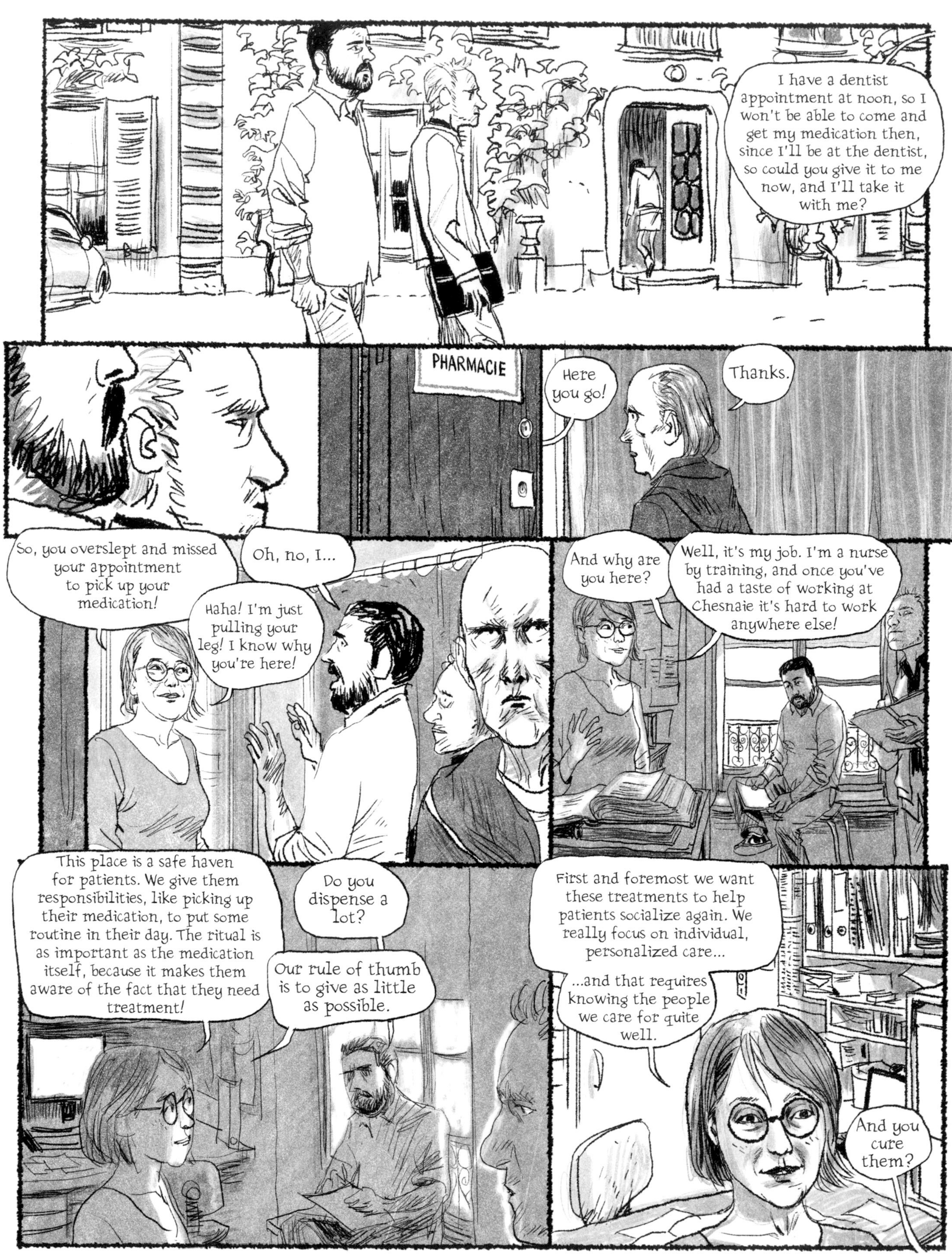
I have a dentist appointment at noon, so I won't be able to come and get my medication then, since I'll be at the dentist, so could you give it to me now, and I'll take it with me?
PHARMACIE
Here you go!
Thanks.
So, you overslept and missed your appointment to pick up your medication!
Oh, no, I...
Haha! I'm just pulling your leg! I know why you're here!
And why are you here?
Well, it's my job. I'm a nurse by training, and once you've had a taste of working at Chesnaie it's hard to work anywhere else!
This place is a safe haven for patients. We give them responsibilities, like picking up their medication, to put some routine in their day. The ritual is as important as the medication itself, because it makes them aware of the fact that they need treatment!
Do you dispense a lot?
Our rule of thumb is to give as little as possible.
First and foremost we want these treatments to help patients socialize again. We really focus on individual, personalized care...
...and that requires knowing the people we care for quite well.
And you cure them?

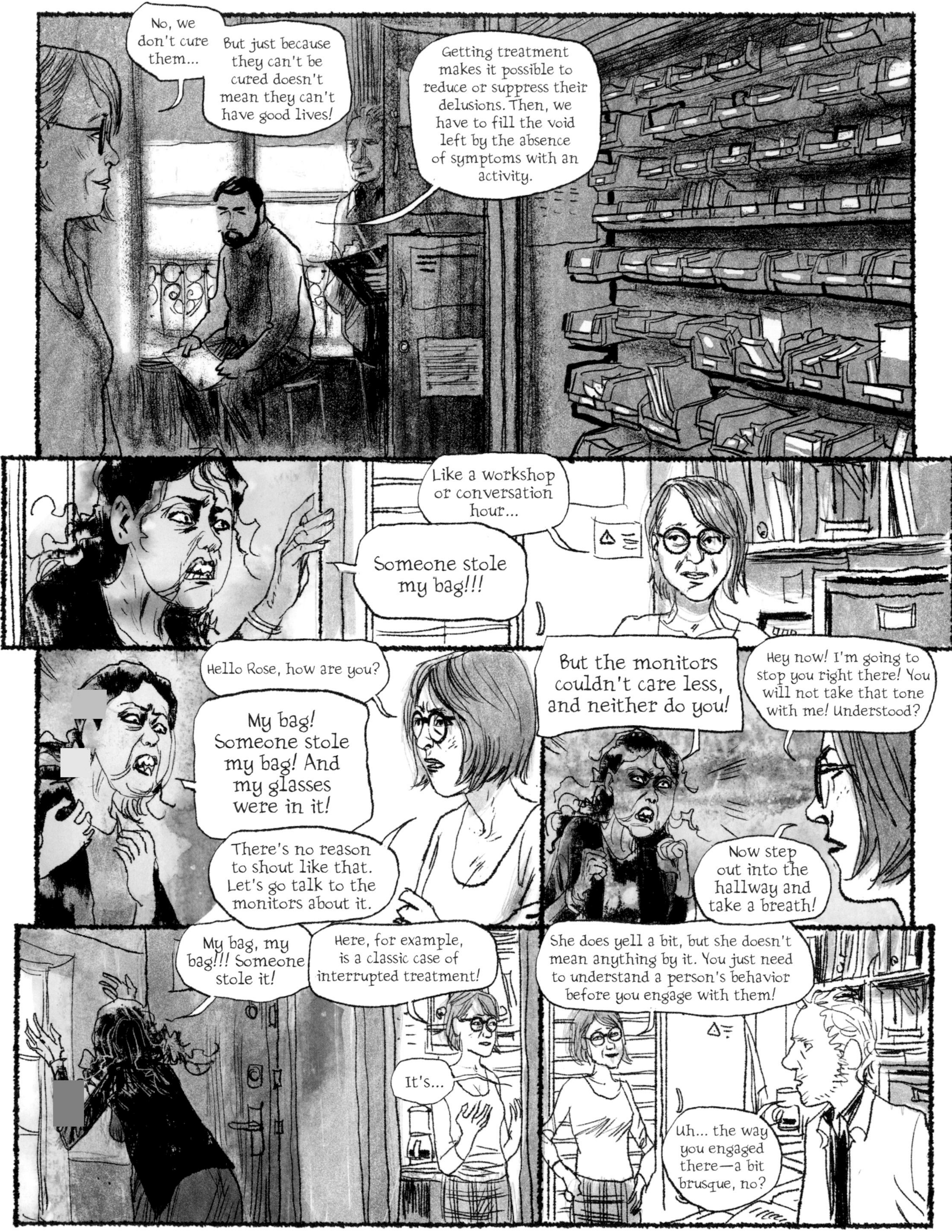
No, we don't cure them...
But just because they can't be cured doesn't mean they can't have good lives!
Getting treatment makes it possible to reduce or suppress their delusions. Then, we have to fill the void left by the absence of symptoms with an activity.
Like a workshop or conversation hour...
Someone stole my bag!!!
Hello Rose, how are you?
My bag! Someone stole my bag! And my glasses were in it!
There's no reason to shout like that. Let's go talk to the monitors about it.
But the monitors couldn't care less, and neither do you!
Hey now! I'm going to stop you right there! You will not take that tone with me! Understood?
Now step out into the hallway and take a breath!
My bag, my bag!!! Someone stole it!
Here, for example, is a classic case of interrupted treatment!
It's...
She does yell a bit, but she doesn't mean anything by it. You just need to understand a person's behavior before you engage with them!
Uh... the way you engaged there—a bit brusque, no?

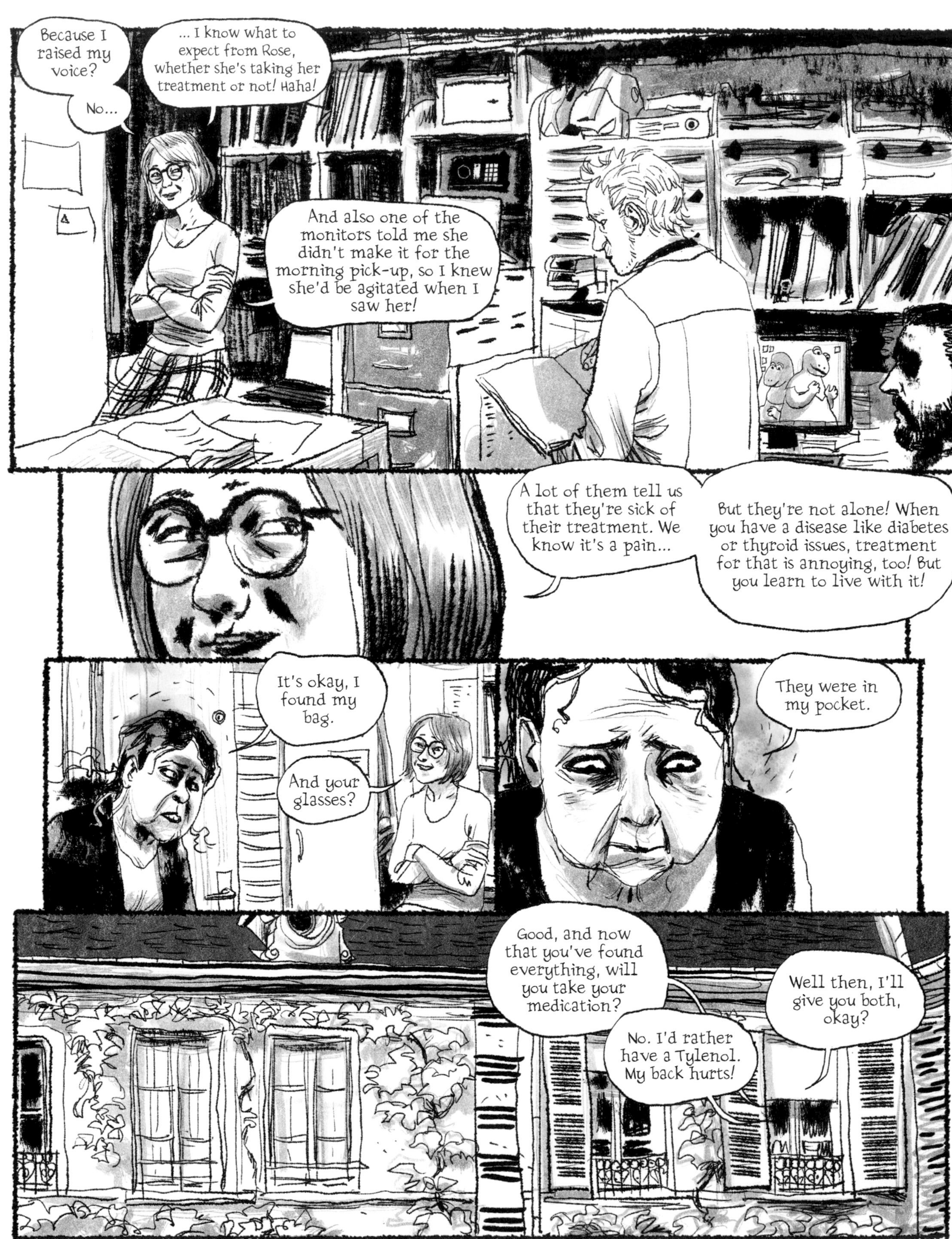
Because I raised my voice?
No...
... I know what to expect from Rose, whether she's taking her treatment or not! Haha!
And also one of the monitors told me she didn't make it for the morning pick-up, so I knew she'd be agitated when I saw her!
A lot of them tell us that they're sick of their treatment. We know it's a pain...
But they're not alone! When you have a disease like diabetes or thyroid issues, treatment for that is annoying, too! But you learn to live with it!
It's okay, I found my bag.
And your glasses?
They were in my pocket.
Good, and now that you've found everything, will you take your medication?
No. I'd rather have a Tylenol. My back hurts!
Well then, I'll give you both, okay?

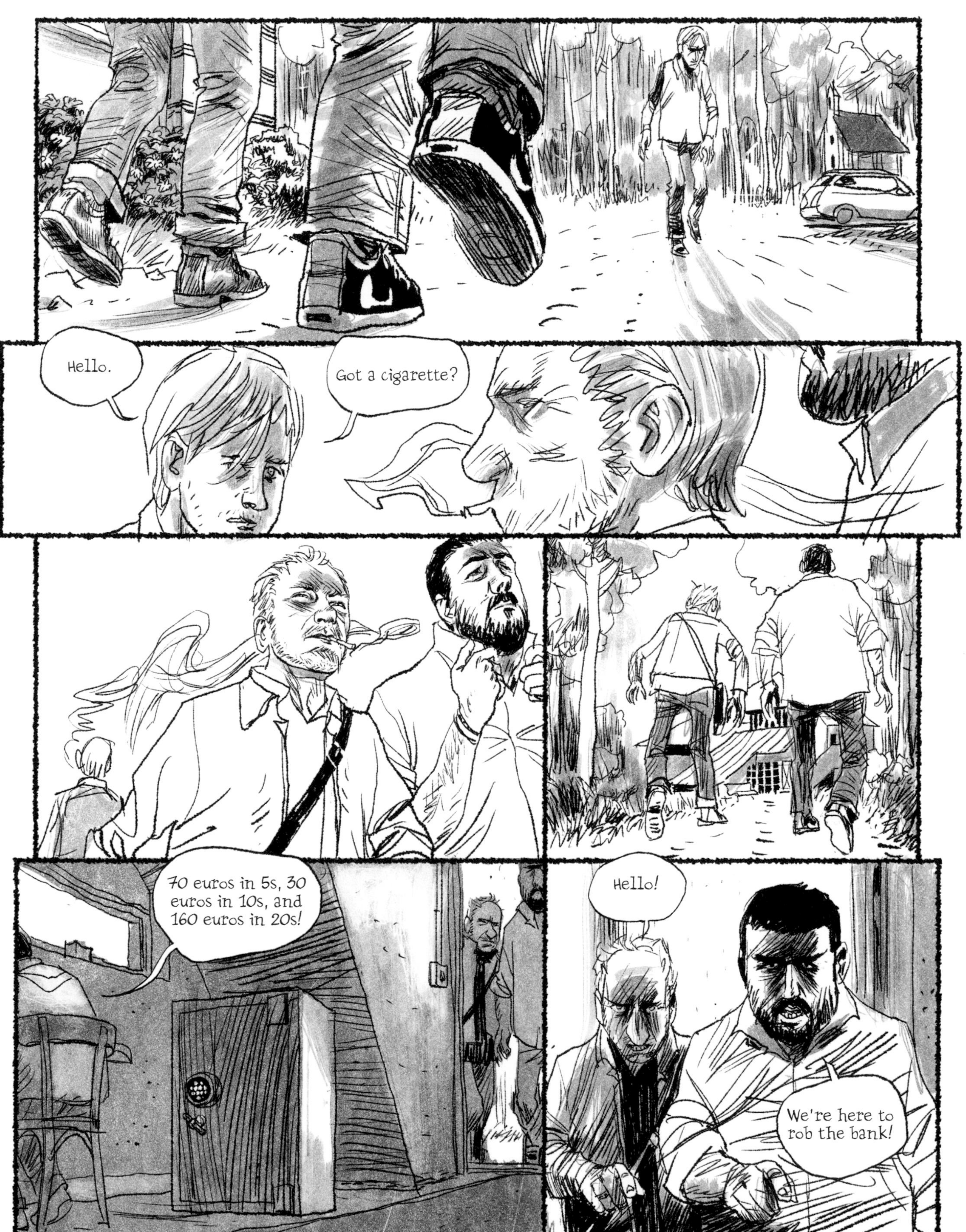
Hello.
Got a cigarette?
70 euros in 5s, 30 euros in 10s, and 160 euros in 20s!
Hello!
We're here to rob the bank!

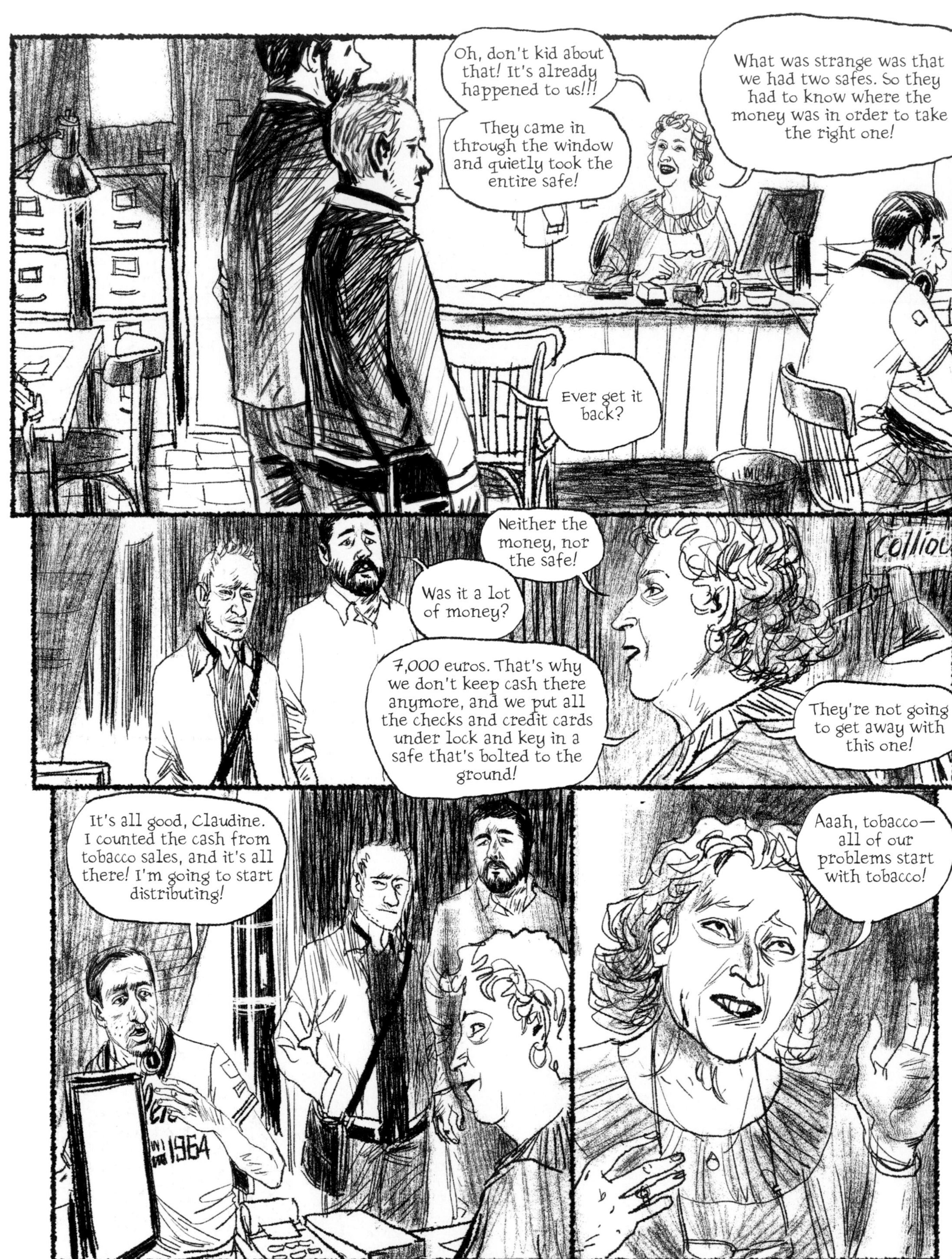
Oh, don't kid about that! It's already happened to us!!!
They came in through the window and quietly took the entire safe!
What was strange was that we had two safes. So they had to know where the money was in order to take the right one!
Ever get it back?
Neither the money, nor the safe!
Was it a lot of money?
7,000 euros. That's why we don't keep cash there anymore, and we put all the checks and credit cards under lock and key in a safe that's bolted to the ground!
They're not going to get away with this one!
It's all good, Claudine. I counted the cash from tobacco sales, and it's all there! I'm going to start distributing!
Aaah, tobacco—all of our problems start with tobacco!

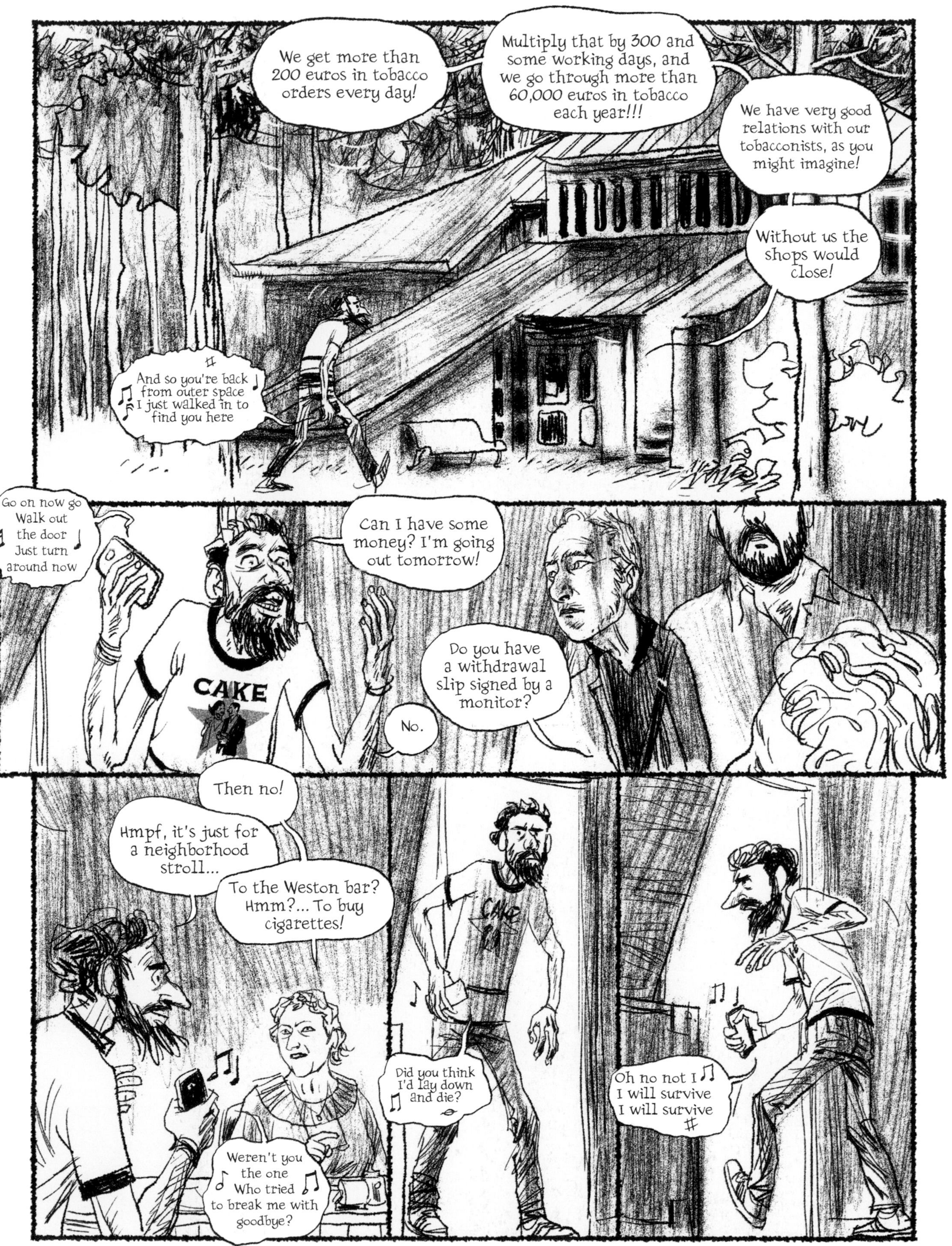
We get more than 200 euros in tobacco orders every day!
Multiply that by 300 and some working days, and we go through more than 60,000 euros in tobacco each year!!!
We have very good relations with our tobacconists, as you might imagine!
Without us the shops would close!
And so you're back from outer space I just walked in to find you here
Go on now go Walk out the door Just turn around now
Can I have some money? I'm going out tomorrow!
Do you have a withdrawal slip signed by a monitor?
No.
CAKE
Then no!
Hmpf, it's just for a neighborhood stroll...
To the Weston bar? Hmm?... To buy cigarettes!
Weren't you the one Who tried to break me with goodbye?
Did you think I'd lay down and die?
Oh no not I I will survive I will survive

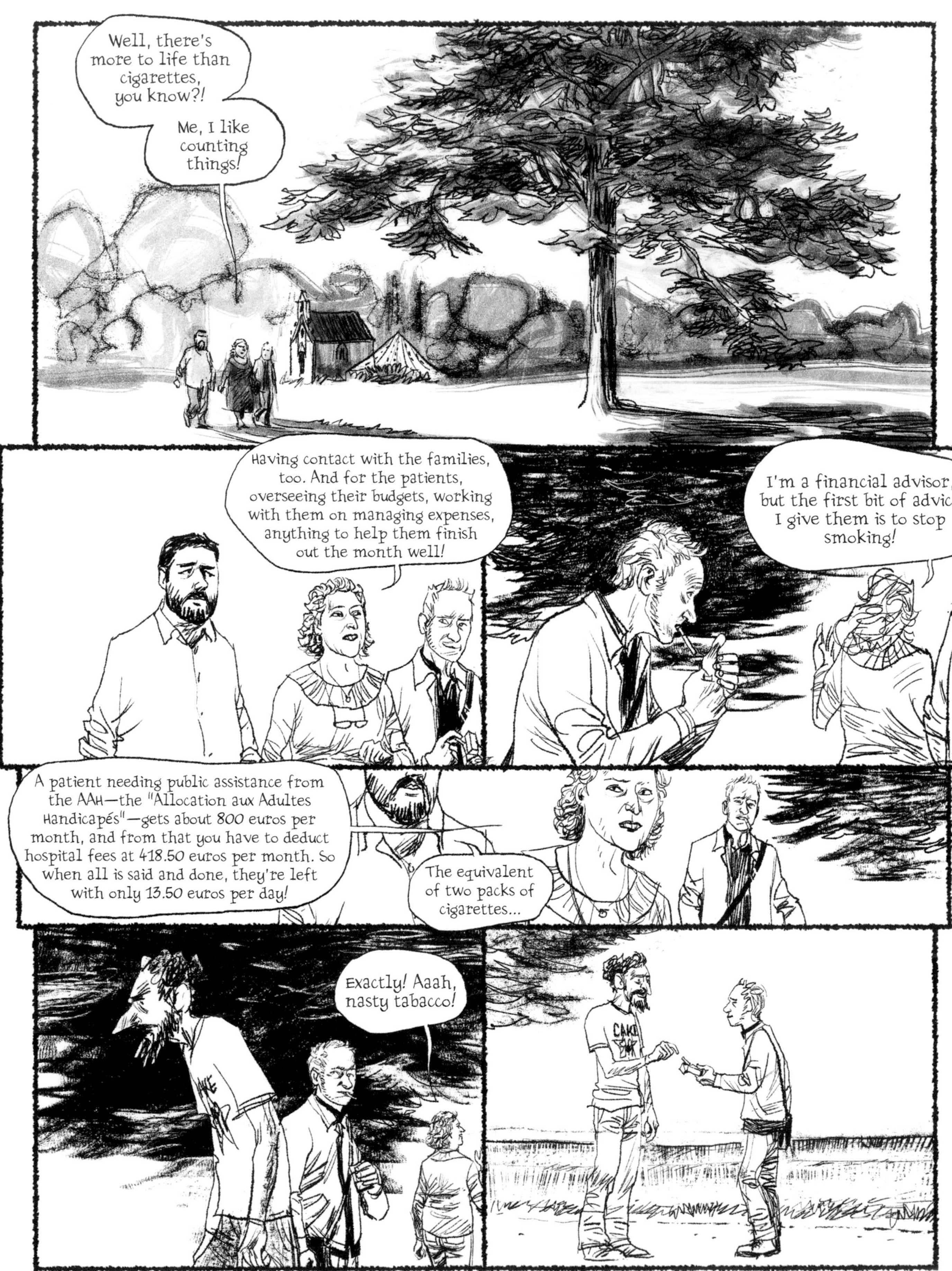
Well, there's more to life than cigarettes, you know?!
Me, I like counting things!
Having contact with the families, too. And for the patients, overseeing their budgets, working with them on managing expenses, anything to help them finish out the month well!
I'm a financial advisor, but the first bit of advice I give them is to stop smoking!
A patient needing public assistance from the AAH—the "Allocation aux Adultes Handicapés"—gets about 800 euros per month, and from that you have to deduct hospital fees at 418.50 euros per month. So when all is said and done, they're left with only 13.50 euros per day!
The equivalent of two packs of cigarettes...
Exactly! Aaah, nasty tabacco!

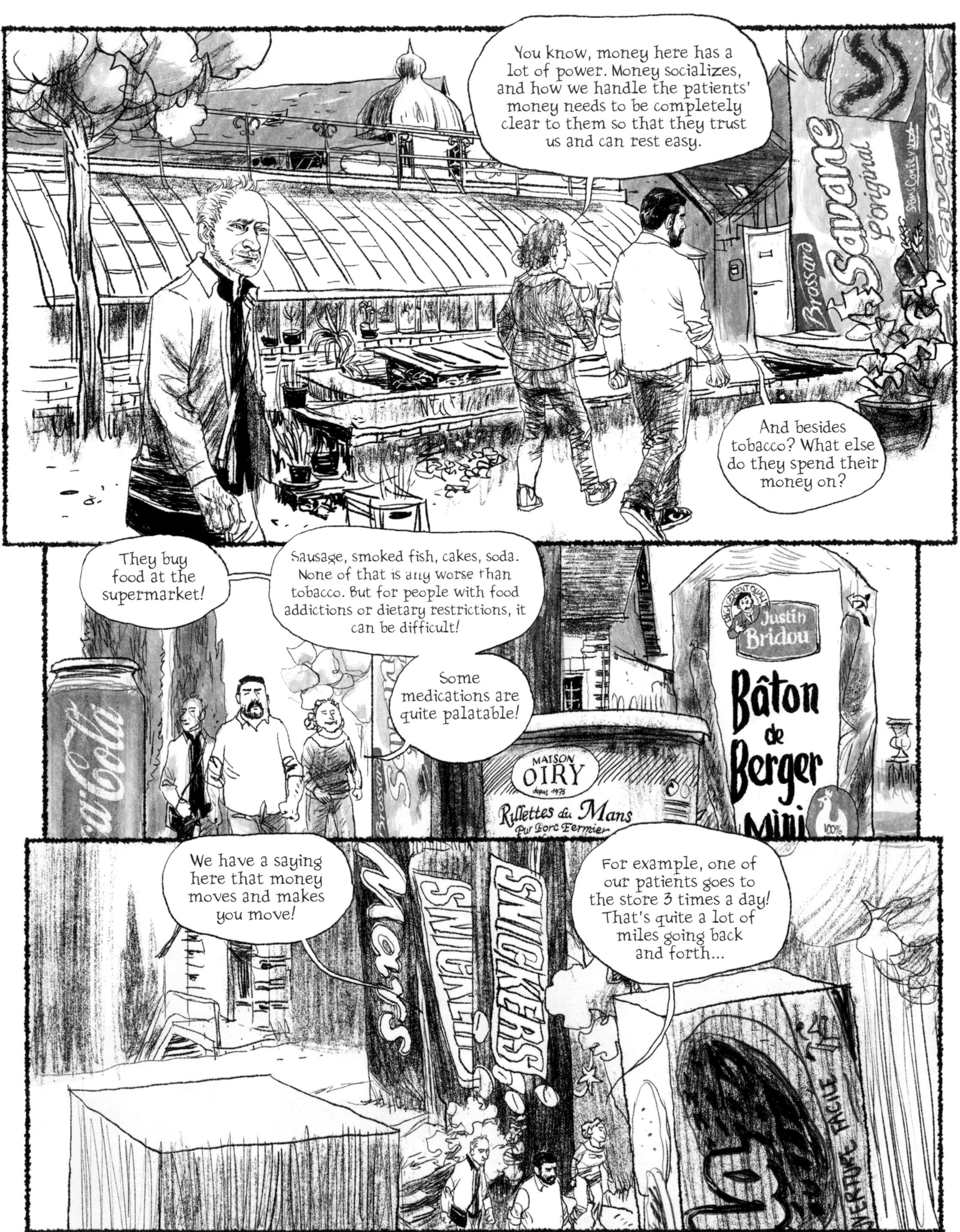
You know, money here has a lot of power. Money socializes, and how we handle the patients' money needs to be completely clear to them so that they trust us and can rest easy.
Brossard
Savane
L'original
And besides tobacco? What else do they spend their money on?
They buy food at the supermarket!
Sausage, smoked fish, cakes, soda. None of that is any worse than tobacco. But for people with food addictions or dietary restrictions, it can be difficult!
Some medications are quite palatable!
Justin Bridou
Bâton de Berger Mini
Maison OIRY
Rillettes du Mans
Pur Porc Fermier
We have a saying here that money moves and makes you move!
Mars
SNICKERS
For example, one of our patients goes to the store 3 times a day! That's quite a lot of miles going back and forth...
OUVERTURE FACILE

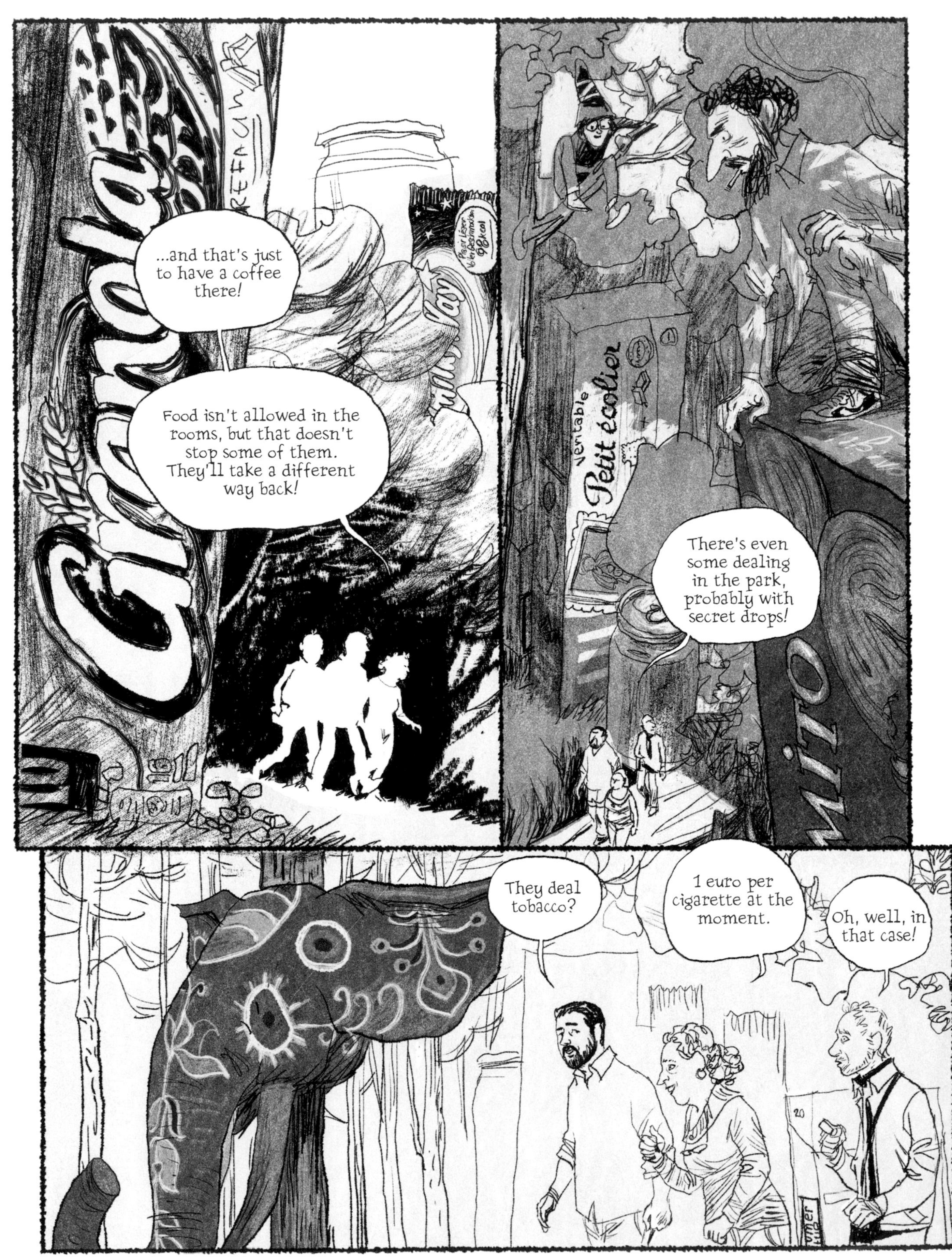
...and that's just to have a coffee there!
Food isn't allowed in the rooms, but that doesn't stop some of them. They'll take a different way back!
There's even some dealing in the park, probably with secret drops!
They deal tobacco?
1 euro per cigarette at the moment.
Oh, well, in that case!

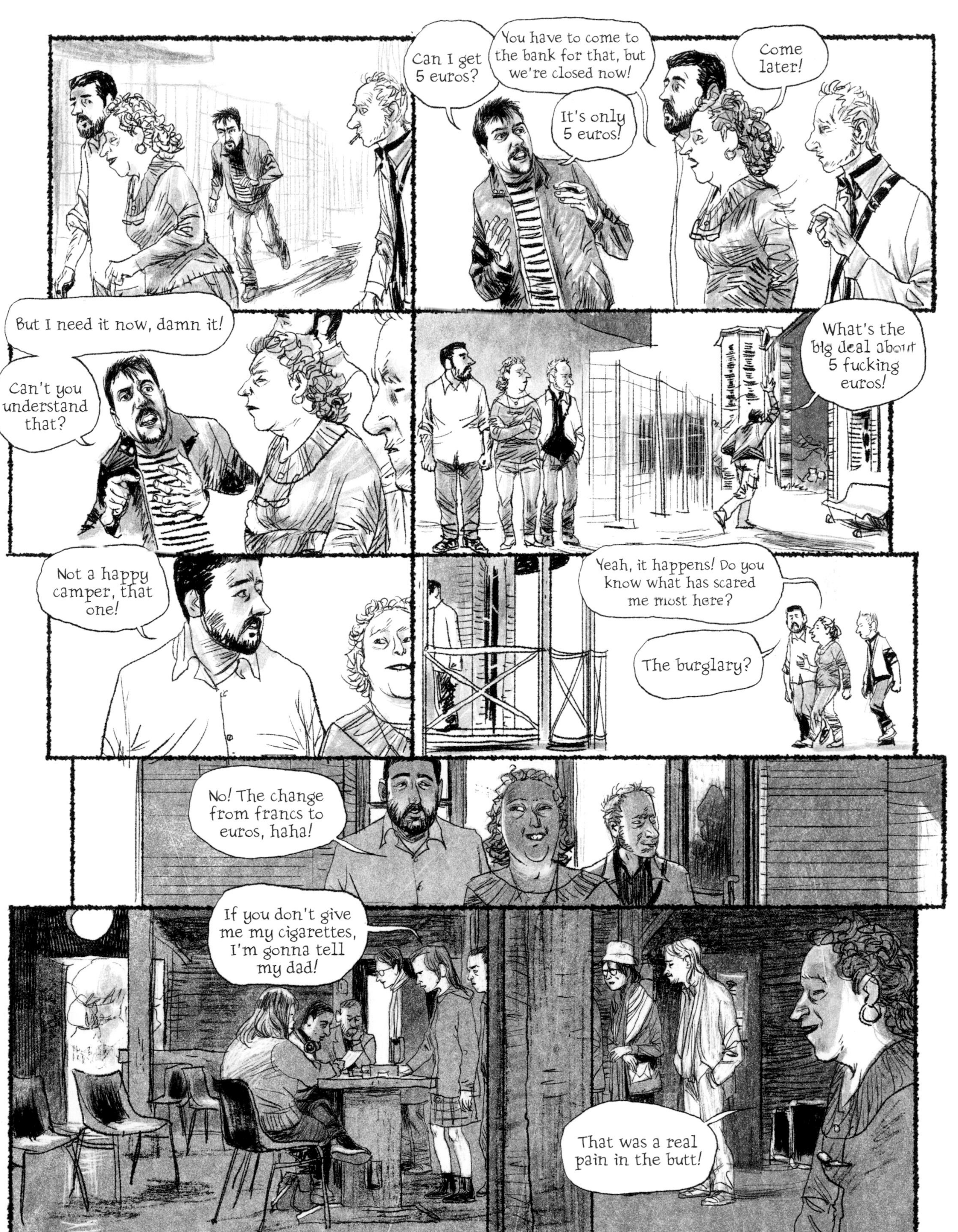
Can I get 5 euros?
You have to come to the bank for that, but we're closed now!
It's only 5 euros!
Come later!
But I need it now, damn it!
Can't you understand that?
What's the big deal about 5 fucking euros!
Not a happy camper, that one!
Yeah, it happens! Do you know what has scared me most here?
The burglary?
No! The change from francs to euros, haha!
If you don't give me my cigarettes, I'm gonna tell my dad!
That was a real pain in the butt!

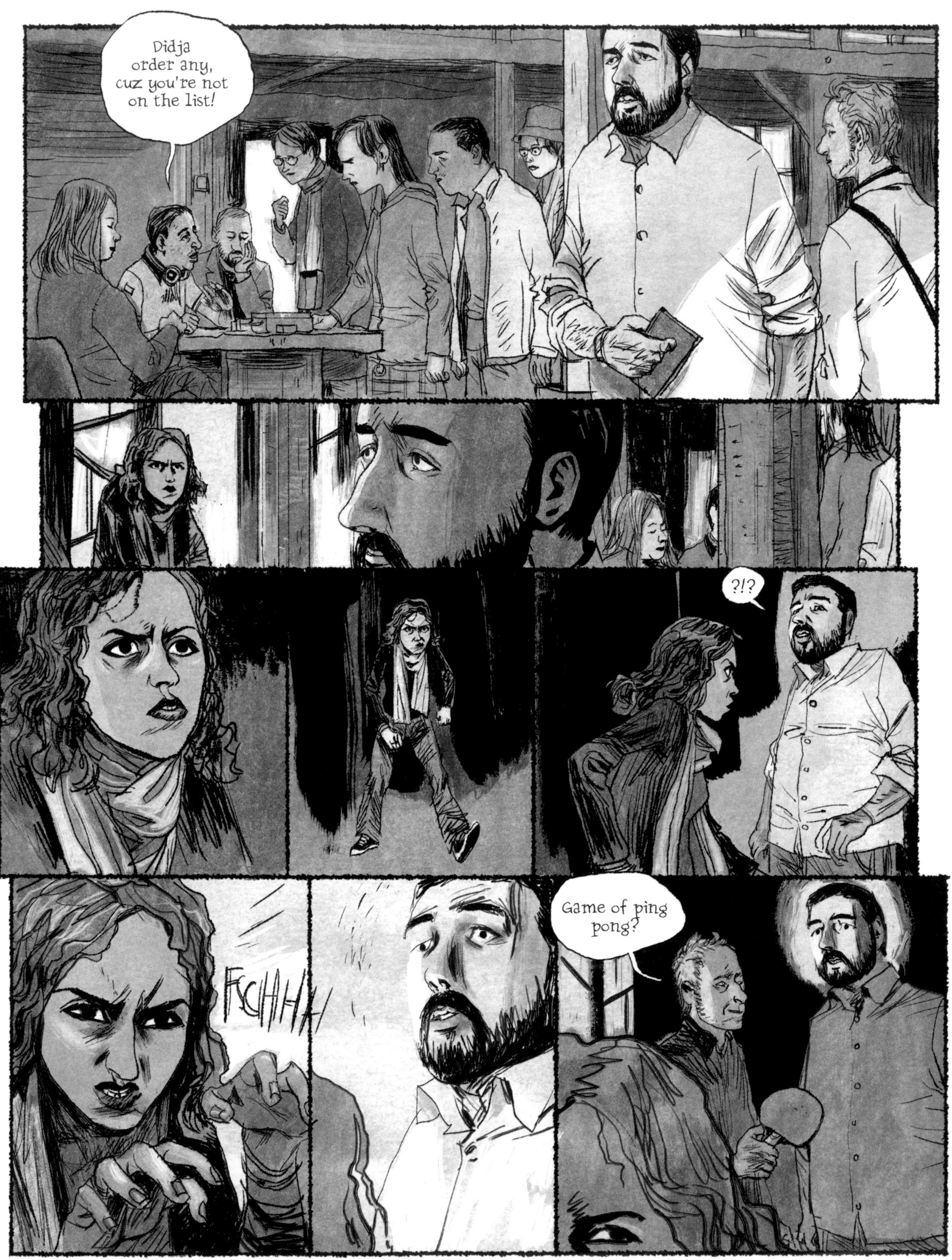
Didja order any, cuz you're not on the list!
?!?
FSCHHH
Game of ping pong?

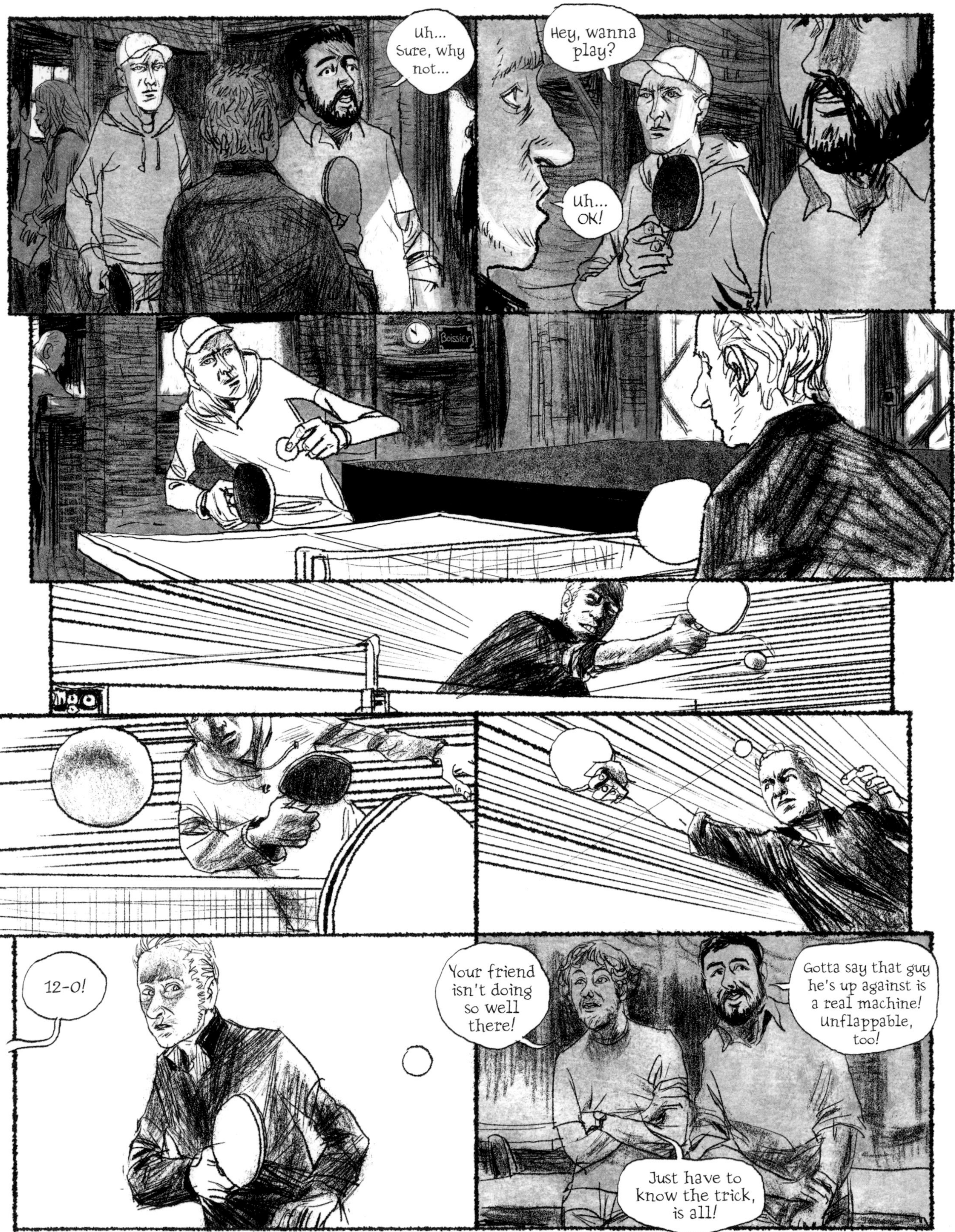
Uh... Sure, why not...
Hey, wanna play?
Uh... OK!
12-0!
Your friend isn't doing so well there!
Gotta say that guy he's up against is a real machine! Unflappable, too!
Just have to know the trick, is all!

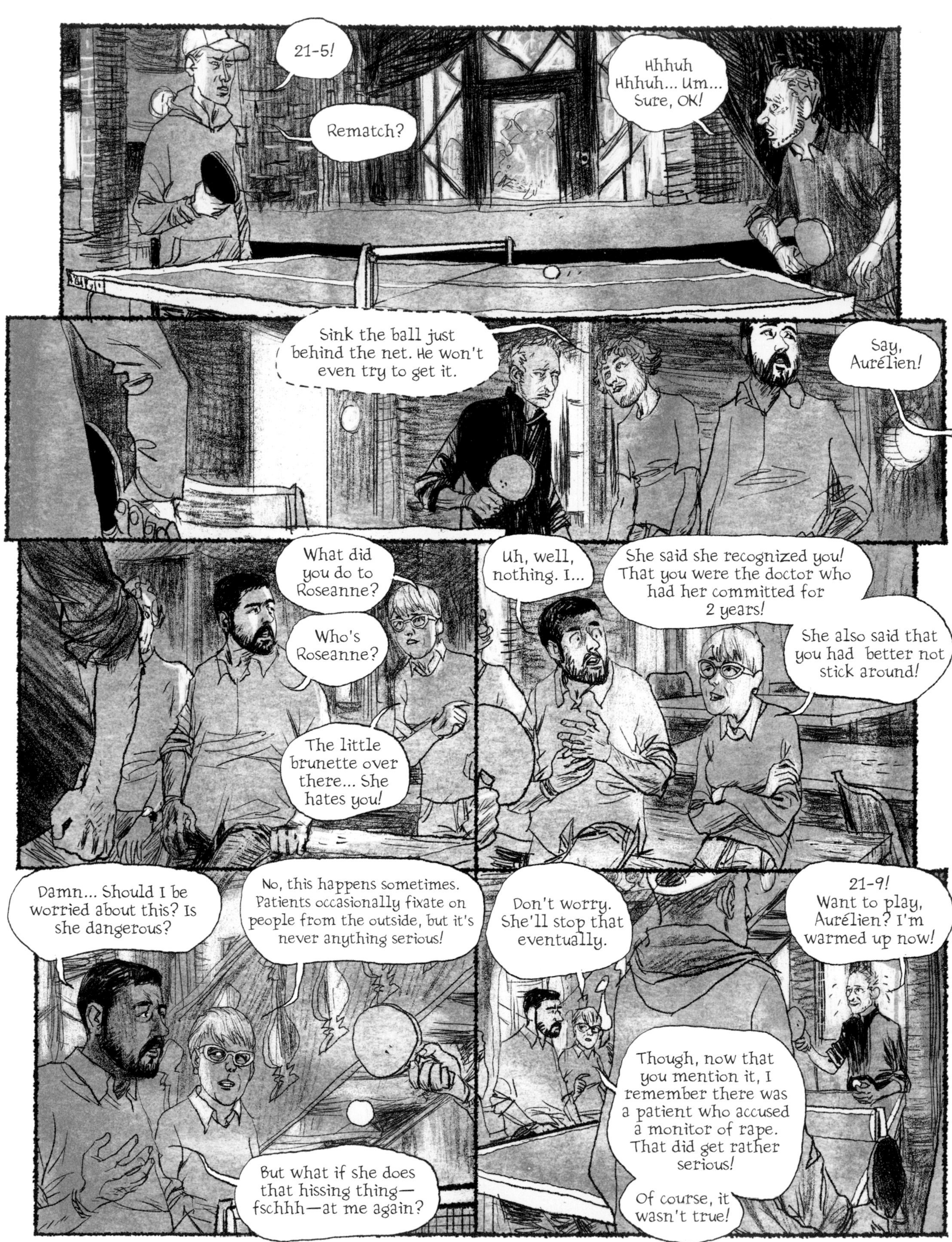
21-5!
Rematch?
Hhhuh Hhhuh... Um... Sure, OK!
Sink the ball just behind the net. He won't even try to get it.
Say, Aurélien!
What did you do to Roseanne?
Who's Roseanne?
The little brunette over there... She hates you!
Uh, well, nothing. I...
She said she recognized you! That you were the doctor who had her committed for 2 years!
She also said that you had better not stick around!
Damn... Should I be worried about this? Is she dangerous?
No, this happens sometimes. Patients occasionally fixate on people from the outside, but it's never anything serious!
But what if she does that hissing thing—fschhh—at me again?
Don't worry. She'll stop that eventually.
21-9! Want to play, Aurélien? I'm warmed up now!
Though, now that you mention it, I remember there was a patient who accused a monitor of rape. That did get rather serious!
Of course, it wasn't true!

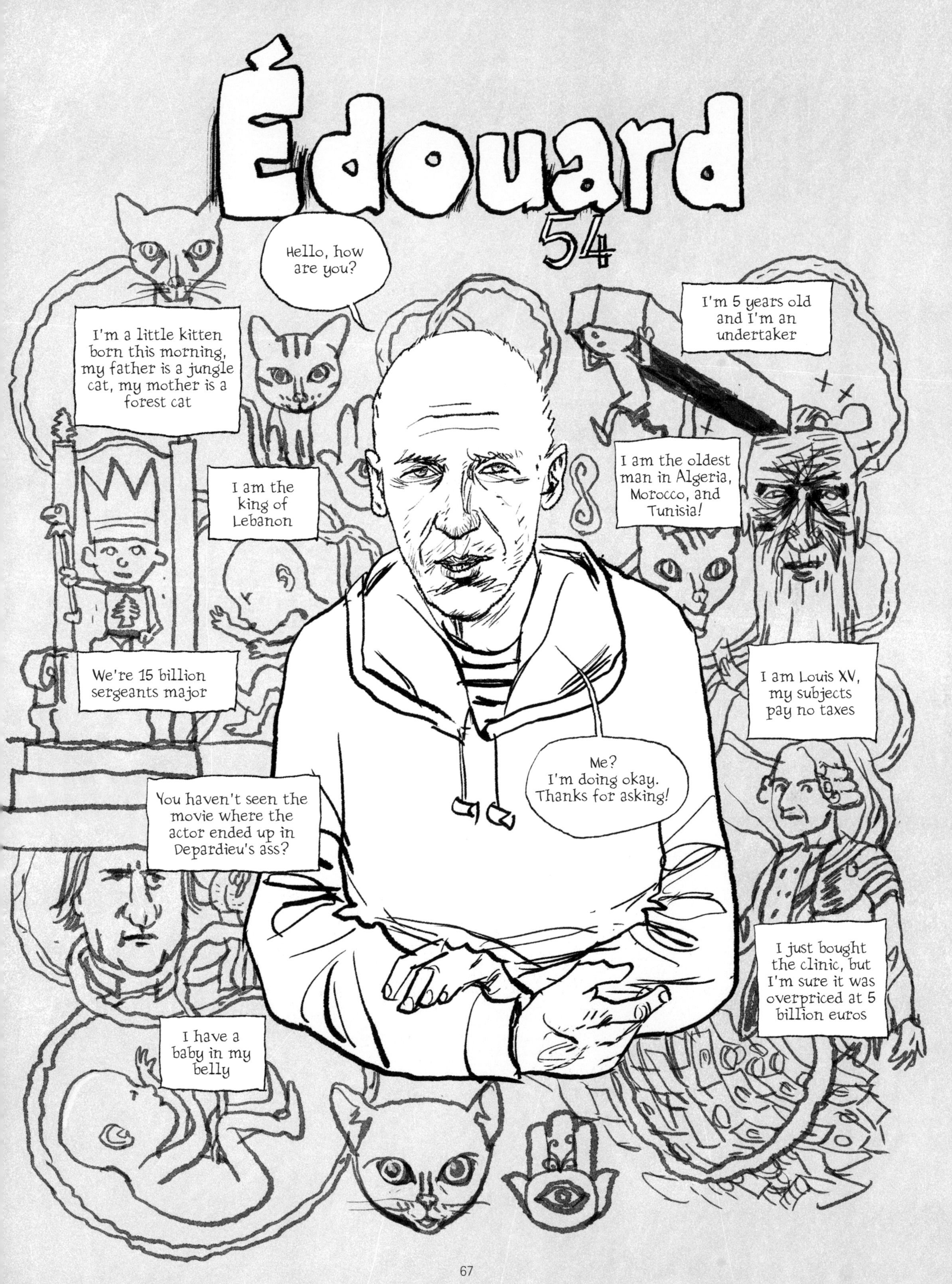
Édouard
54
Hello, how are you?
I'm a little kitten born this morning, my father is a jungle cat, my mother is a forest cat
I am the king of Lebanon
We're 15 billion sergeants major
You haven't seen the movie where the actor ended up in Depardieu's ass?
I have a baby in my belly
I'm 5 years old and I'm an undertaker
I am the oldest man in Algeria, Morocco, and Tunisia!
I am Louis XV, my subjects pay no taxes
Me? I'm doing okay. Thanks for asking!
I just bought the clinic, but I'm sure it was overpriced at 5 billion euros

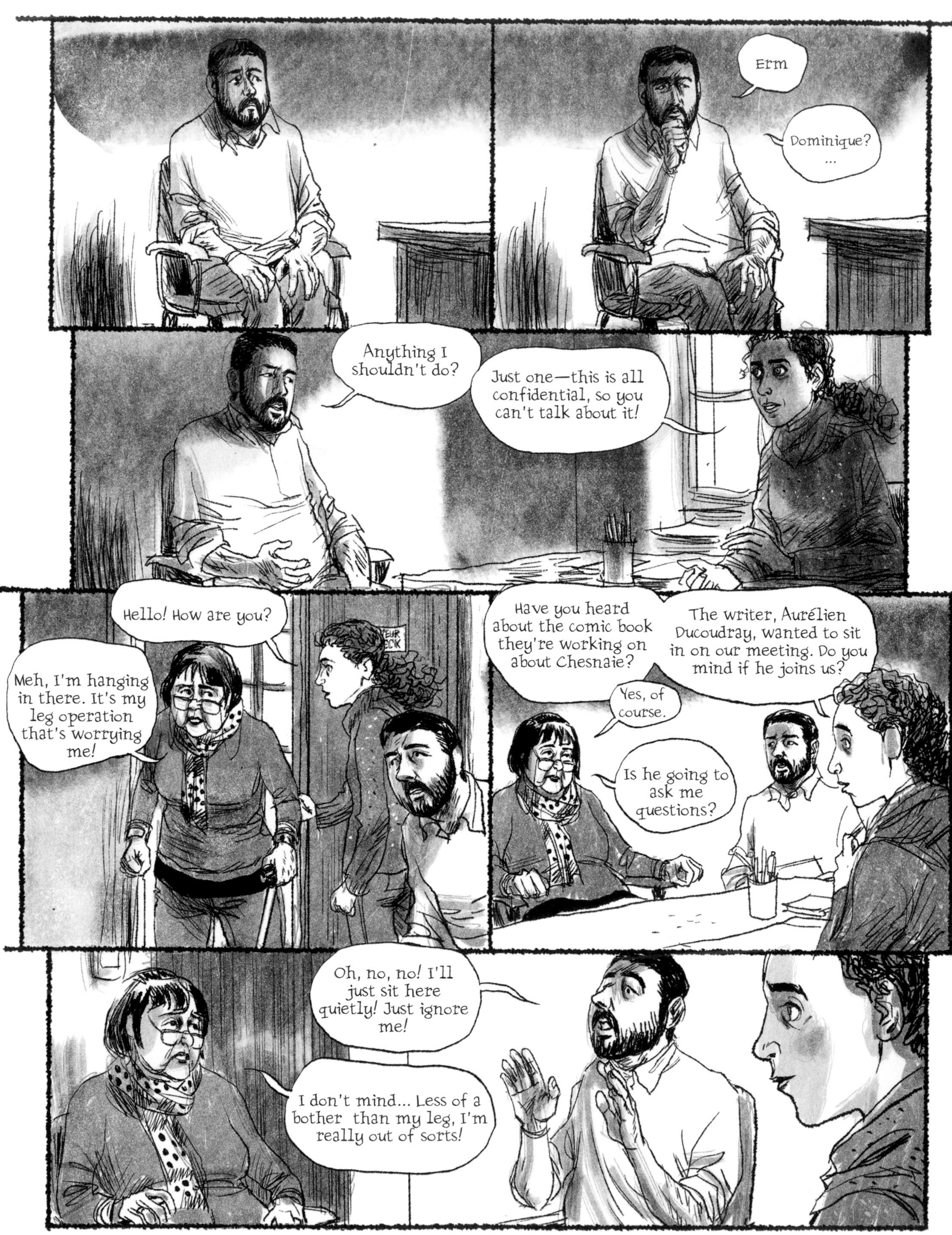
Erm
Dominique? ...
Anything I shouldn't do?
Just one—this is all confidential, so you can't talk about it!
Hello! How are you?
Meh, I'm hanging in there. It's my leg operation that's worrying me!
Have you heard about the comic book they're working on about Chesnaie?
The writer, Aurélien Ducoudray, wanted to sit in on our meeting. Do you mind if he joins us?
Yes, of course.
Is he going to ask me questions?
Oh, no, no! I'll just sit here quietly! Just ignore me!
I don't mind... Less of a bother than my leg, I'm really out of sorts!

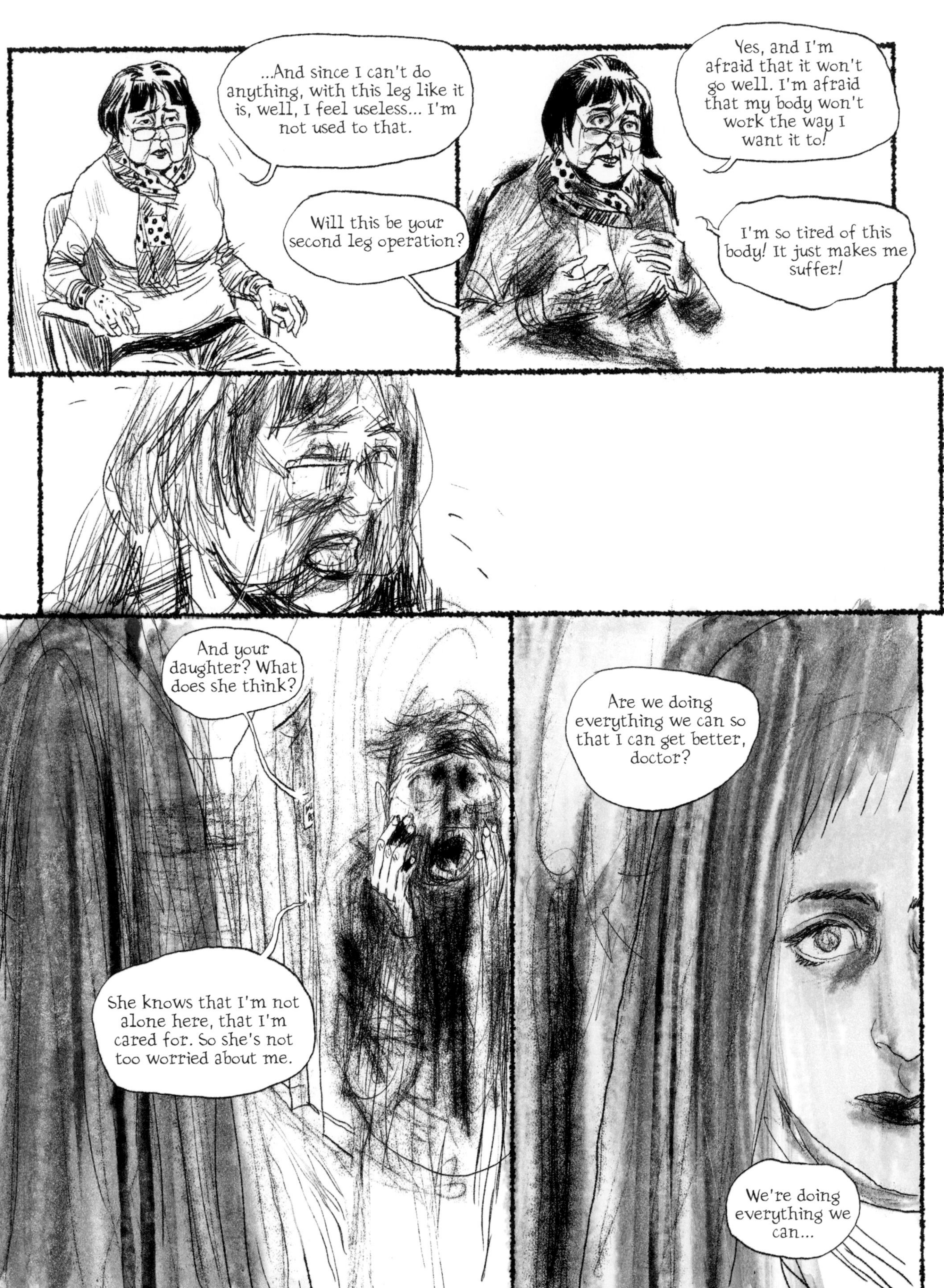
...And since I can't do anything, with this leg like it is, well, I feel useless... I'm not used to that.
Will this be your second leg operation?
Yes, and I'm afraid that it won't go well. I'm afraid that my body won't work the way I want it to!
I'm so tired of this body! It just makes me suffer!
And your daughter? What does she think?
She knows that I'm not alone here, that I'm cared for. So she's not too worried about me.
Are we doing everything we can so that I can get better, doctor?
We're doing everything we can...

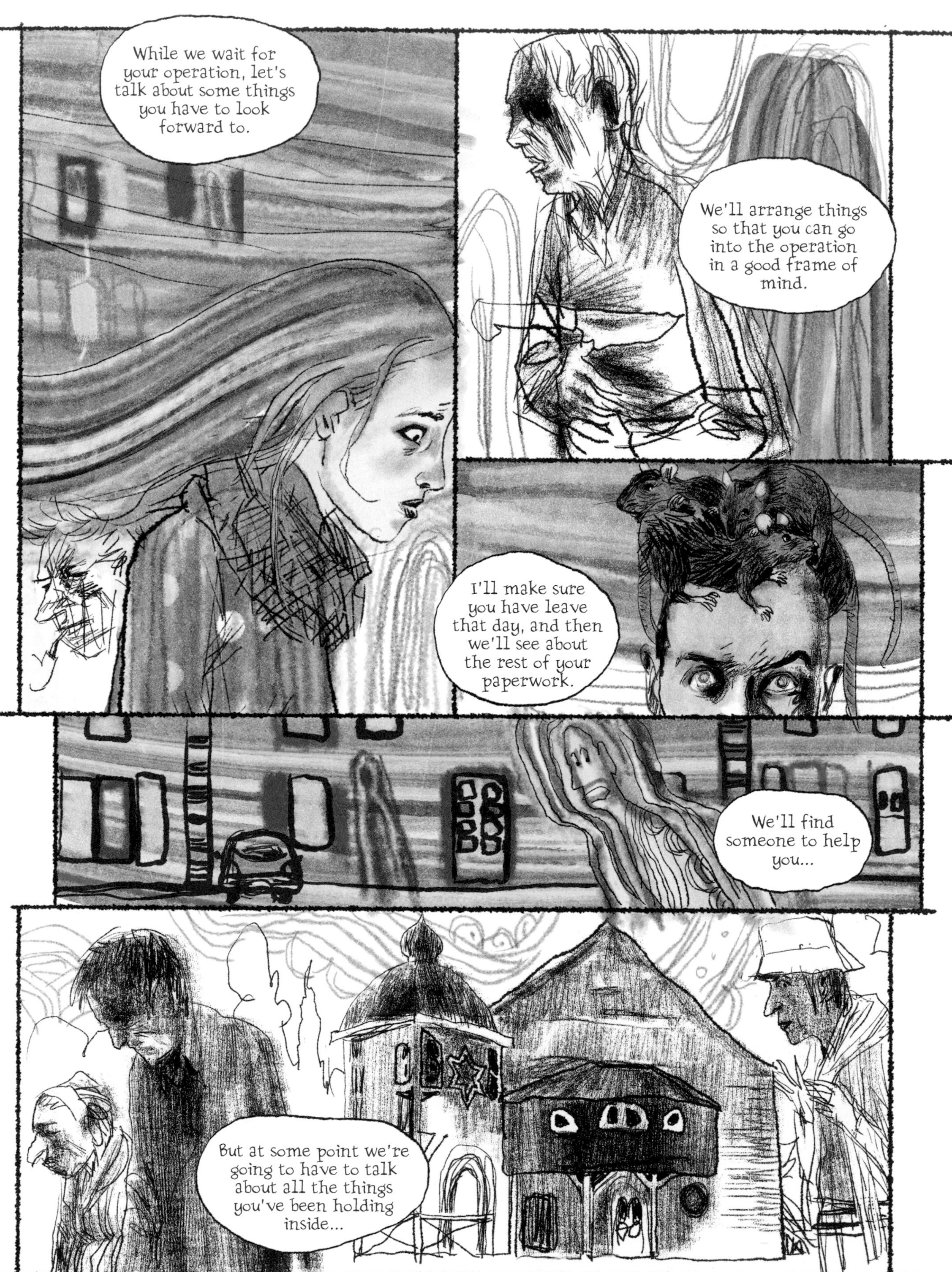
While we wait for your operation, let's talk about some things you have to look forward to.
We'll arrange things so that you can go into the operation in a good frame of mind.
I'll make sure you have leave that day, and then we'll see about the rest of your paperwork.
We'll find someone to help you...
But at some point we're going to have to talk about all the things you've been holding inside...

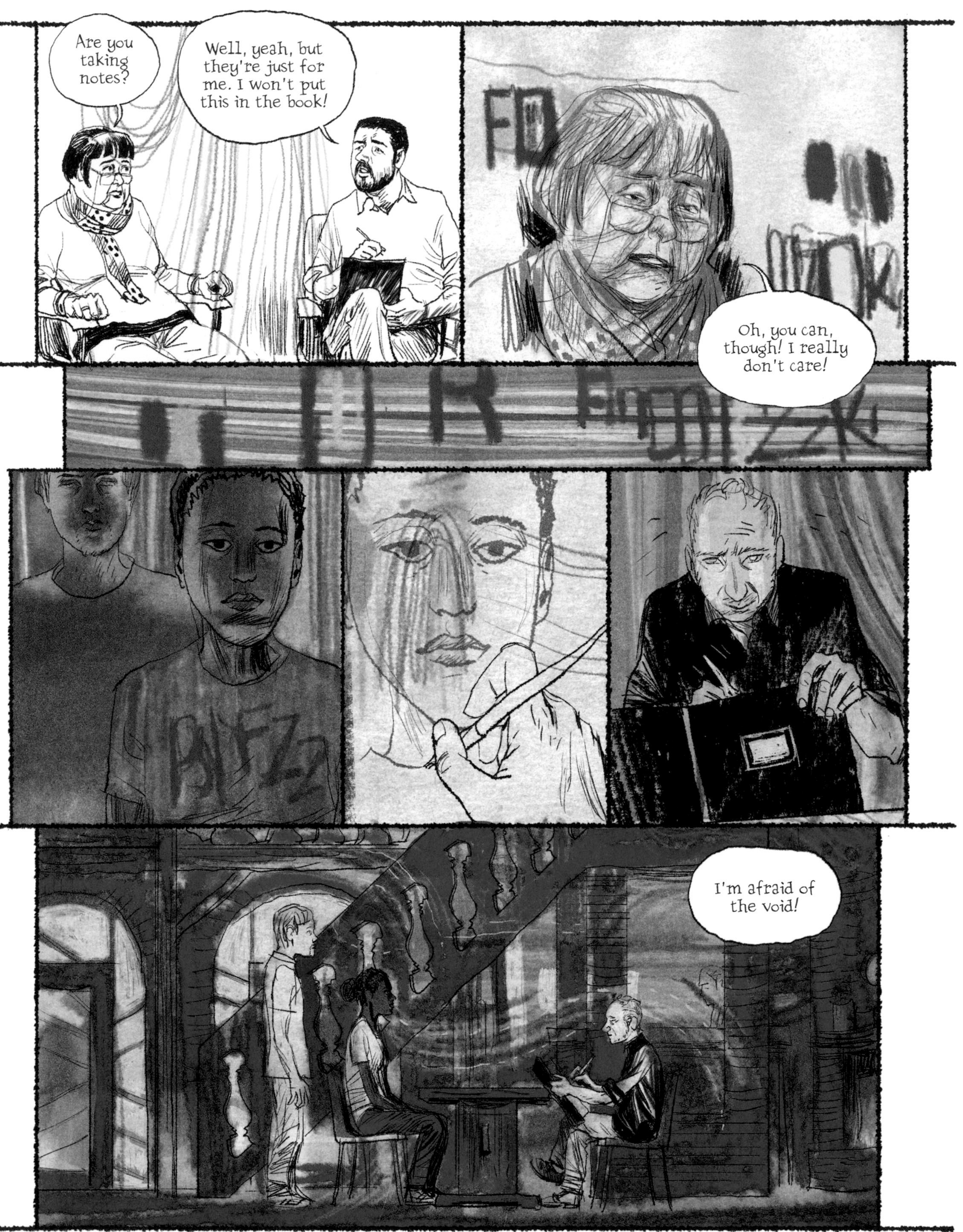
Are you taking notes?
Well, yeah, but they're just for me. I won't put this in the book!
Oh, you can, though! I really don't care!
I'm afraid of the void!

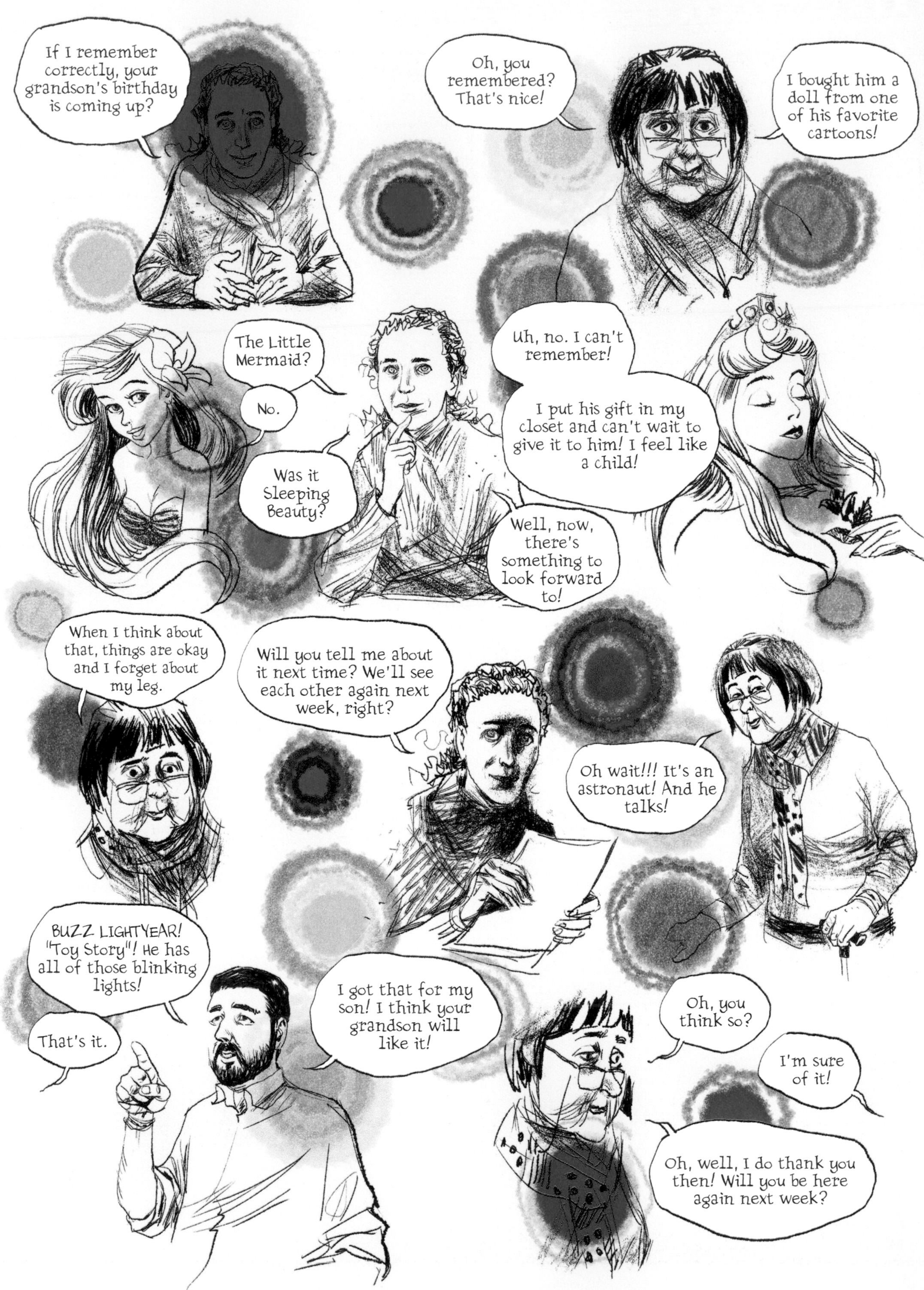
If I remember correctly, your grandson's birthday is coming up?
Oh, you remembered? That's nice!
I bought him a doll from one of his favorite cartoons!
The Little Mermaid?
No.
Was it Sleeping Beauty?
Uh, no. I can't remember!
I put his gift in my closet and can't wait to give it to him! I feel like a child!
Well, now, there's something to look forward to!
When I think about that, things are okay and I forget about my leg.
Will you tell me about it next time? We'll see each other again next week, right?
Oh wait!!! It's an astronaut! And he talks!
BUZZ LIGHTYEAR! "Toy Story"! He has all of those blinking lights!
That's it.
I got that for my son! I think your grandson will like it!
Oh, you think so?
I'm sure of it!
Oh, well, I do thank you then! Will you be here again next week?

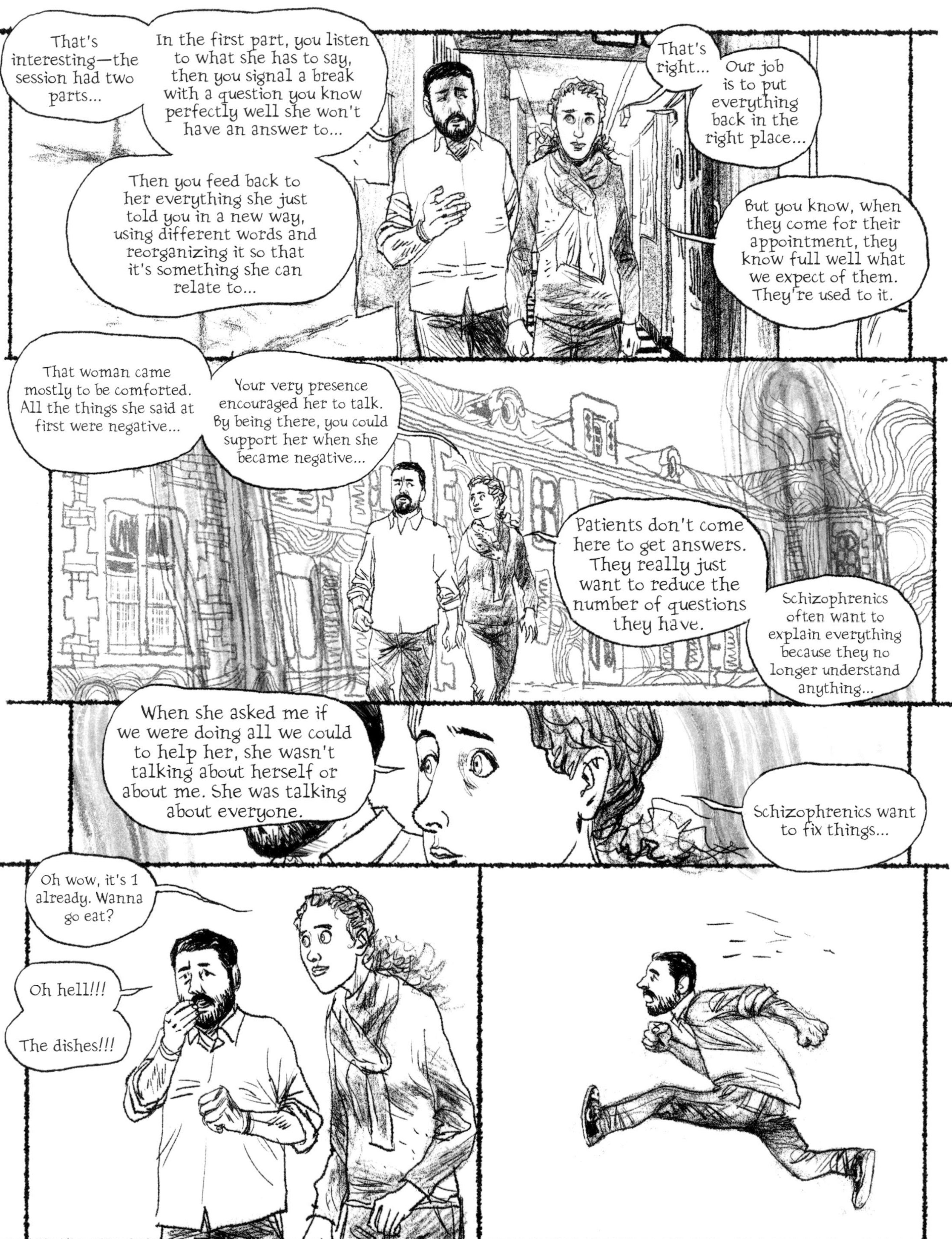
That's interesting—the session had two parts...
In the first part, you listen to what she has to say, then you signal a break with a question you know perfectly well she won't have an answer to...
Then you feed back to her everything she just told you in a new way, using different words and reorganizing it so that it's something she can relate to...
That's right...
Our job is to put everything back in the right place...
But you know, when they come for their appointment, they know full well what we expect of them. They're used to it.
That woman came mostly to be comforted. All the things she said at first were negative...
Your very presence encouraged her to talk. By being there, you could support her when she became negative...
Patients don't come here to get answers. They really just want to reduce the number of questions they have.
Schizophrenics often want to explain everything because they no longer understand anything...
When she asked me if we were doing all we could to help her, she wasn't talking about herself or about me. She was talking about everyone.
Schizophrenics want to fix things...
Oh wow, it's 1 already. Wanna go eat?
Oh hell!!!
The dishes!!!

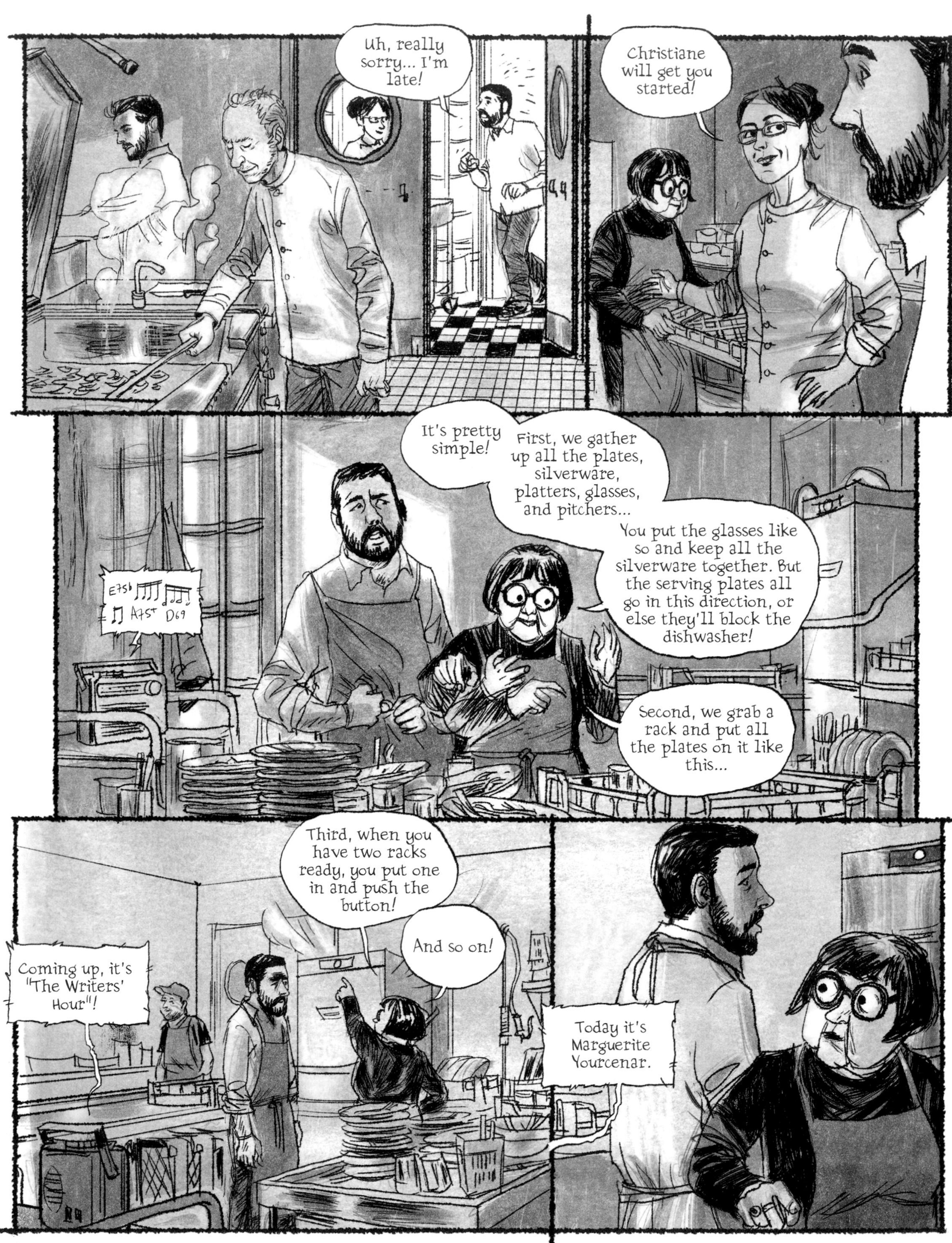
Uh, really sorry... I'm late!
Christiane will get you started!
It's pretty simple!
First, we gather up all the plates, silverware, platters, glasses, and pitchers...
You put the glasses like so and keep all the silverware together. But the serving plates all go in this direction, or else they'll block the dishwasher!
Second, we grab a rack and put all the plates on it like this...
Third, when you have two racks ready, you put one in and push the button!
And so on!
Coming up, it's "The Writers' Hour"!
Today it's Marguerite Yourcenar.

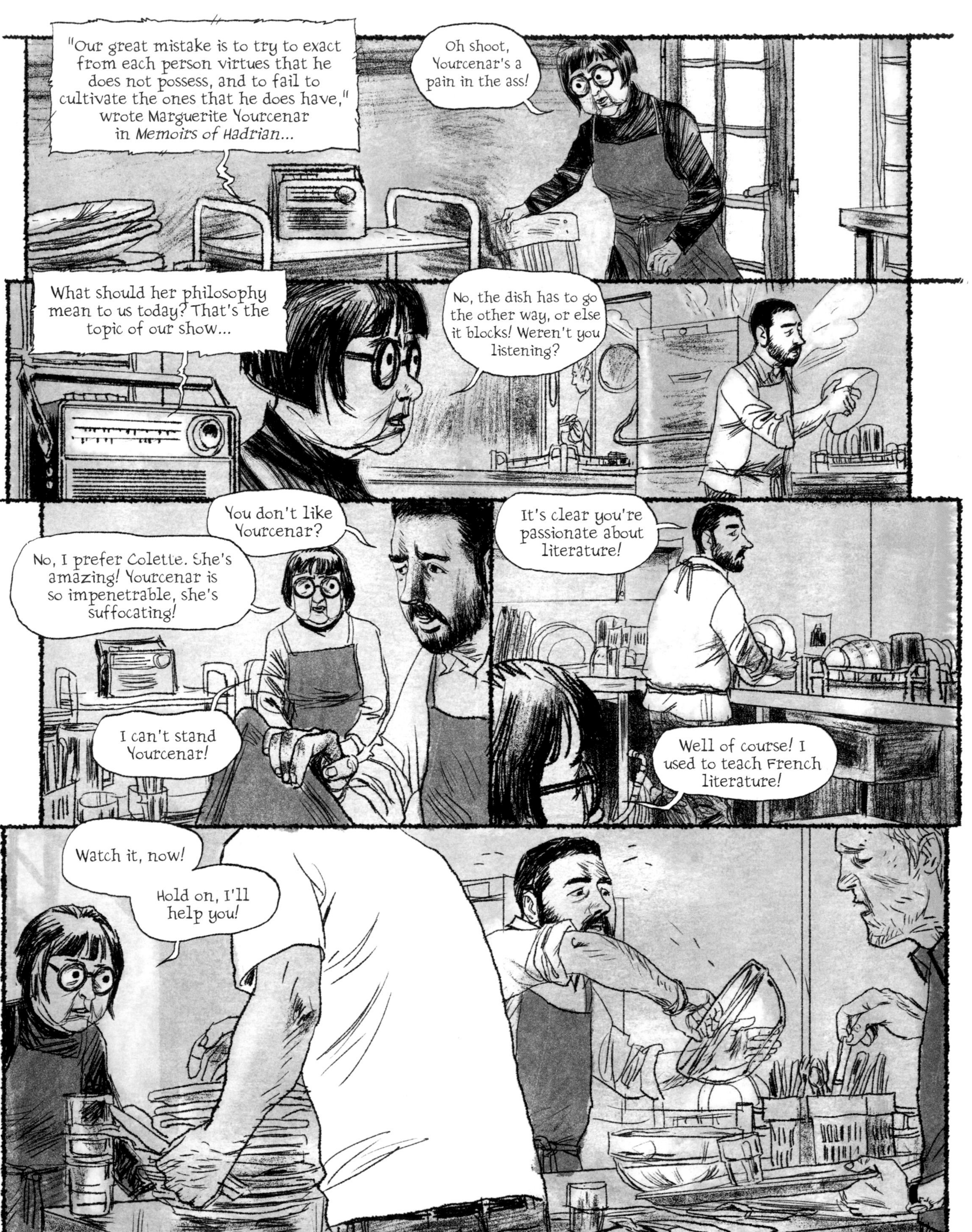
"Our great mistake is to try to exact from each person virtues that he does not possess, and to fail to cultivate the ones that he does have," wrote Marguerite Yourcenar in *Memoirs of Hadrian*...
Oh shoot, Yourcenar's a pain in the ass!
What should her philosophy mean to us today? That's the topic of our show...
No, the dish has to go the other way, or else it blocks! Weren't you listening?
You don't like Yourcenar?
No, I prefer Colette. She's amazing! Yourcenar is so impenetrable, she's suffocating!
I can't stand Yourcenar!
It's clear you're passionate about literature!
Well of course! I used to teach French literature!
Watch it, now!
Hold on, I'll help you!

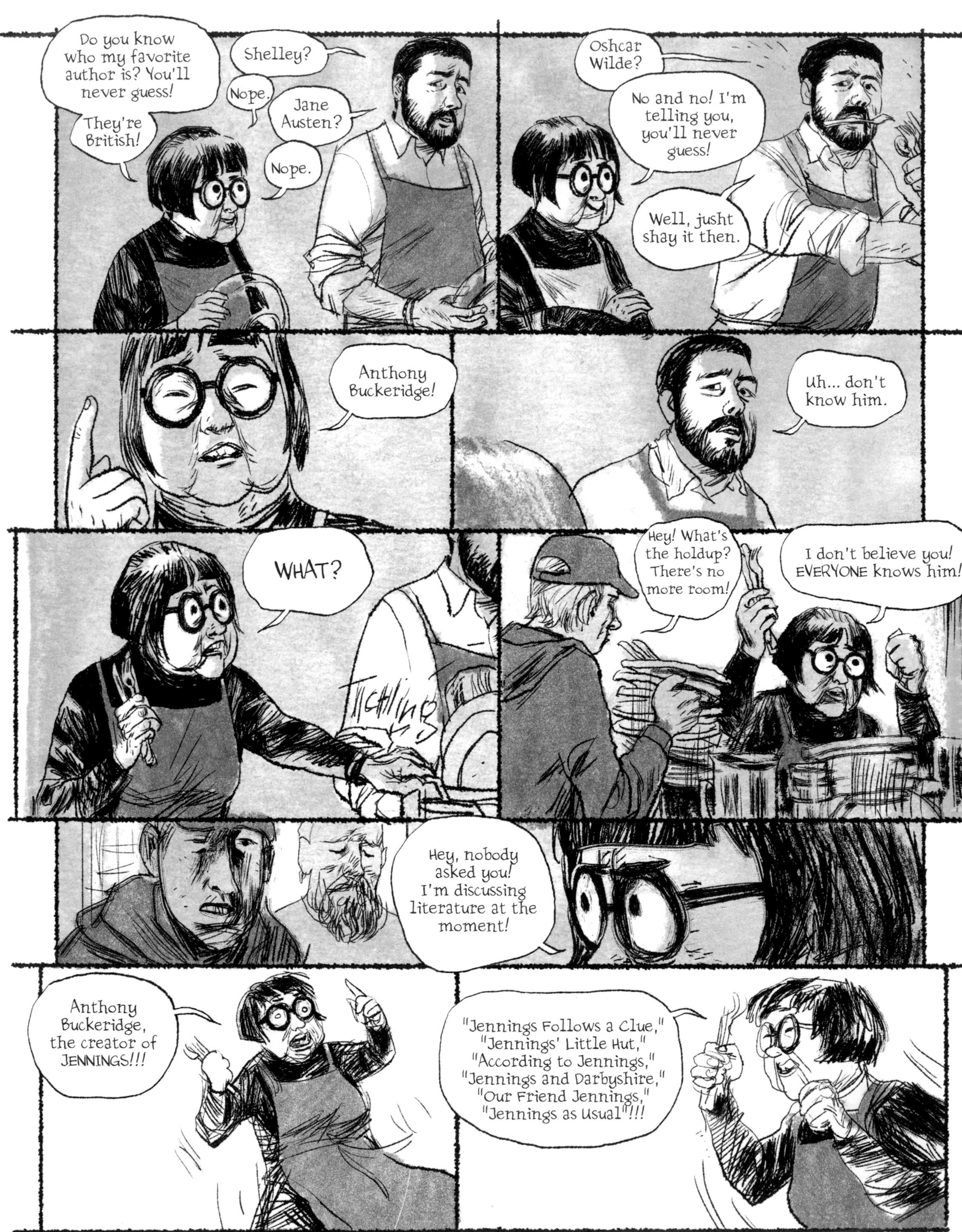
Do you know who my favorite author is? You'll never guess!
They're British!
Shelley?
Nope.
Jane Austen?
Nope.
Oshcar Wilde?
No and no! I'm telling you, you'll never guess!
Well, jusht shay it then.
Anthony Buckeridge!
Uh... don't know him.
WHAT?
Tichling
Hey! What's the holdup? There's no more room!
I don't believe you! EVERYONE knows him!
Hey, nobody asked you! I'm discussing literature at the moment!
Anthony Buckeridge, the creator of JENNINGS!!!
"Jennings Follows a Clue," "Jennings' Little Hut," "According to Jennings," "Jennings and Darbyshire," "Our Friend Jennings," "Jennings as Usual"!!!

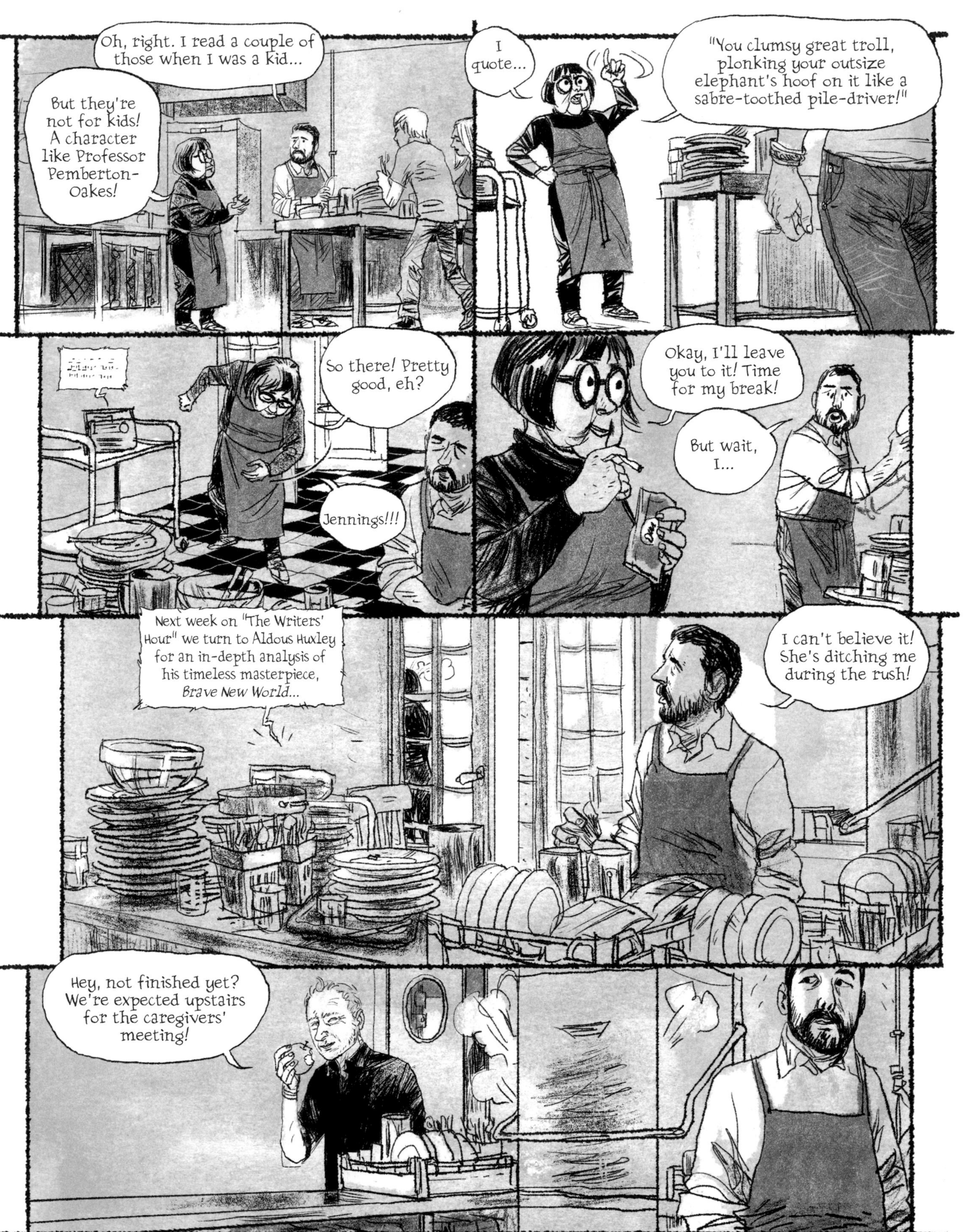
Oh, right. I read a couple of those when I was a kid...
But they're not for kids! A character like Professor Pemberton-Oakes!
I quote...
"You clumsy great troll, plonking your outsize elephant's hoof on it like a sabre-toothed pile-driver!"
So there! Pretty good, eh?
Jennings!!!
Okay, I'll leave you to it! Time for my break!
But wait, I...
Next week on "The Writers' Hour" we turn to Aldous Huxley for an in-depth analysis of his timeless masterpiece, *Brave New World*...
I can't believe it! She's ditching me during the rush!
Hey, not finished yet? We're expected upstairs for the caregivers' meeting!

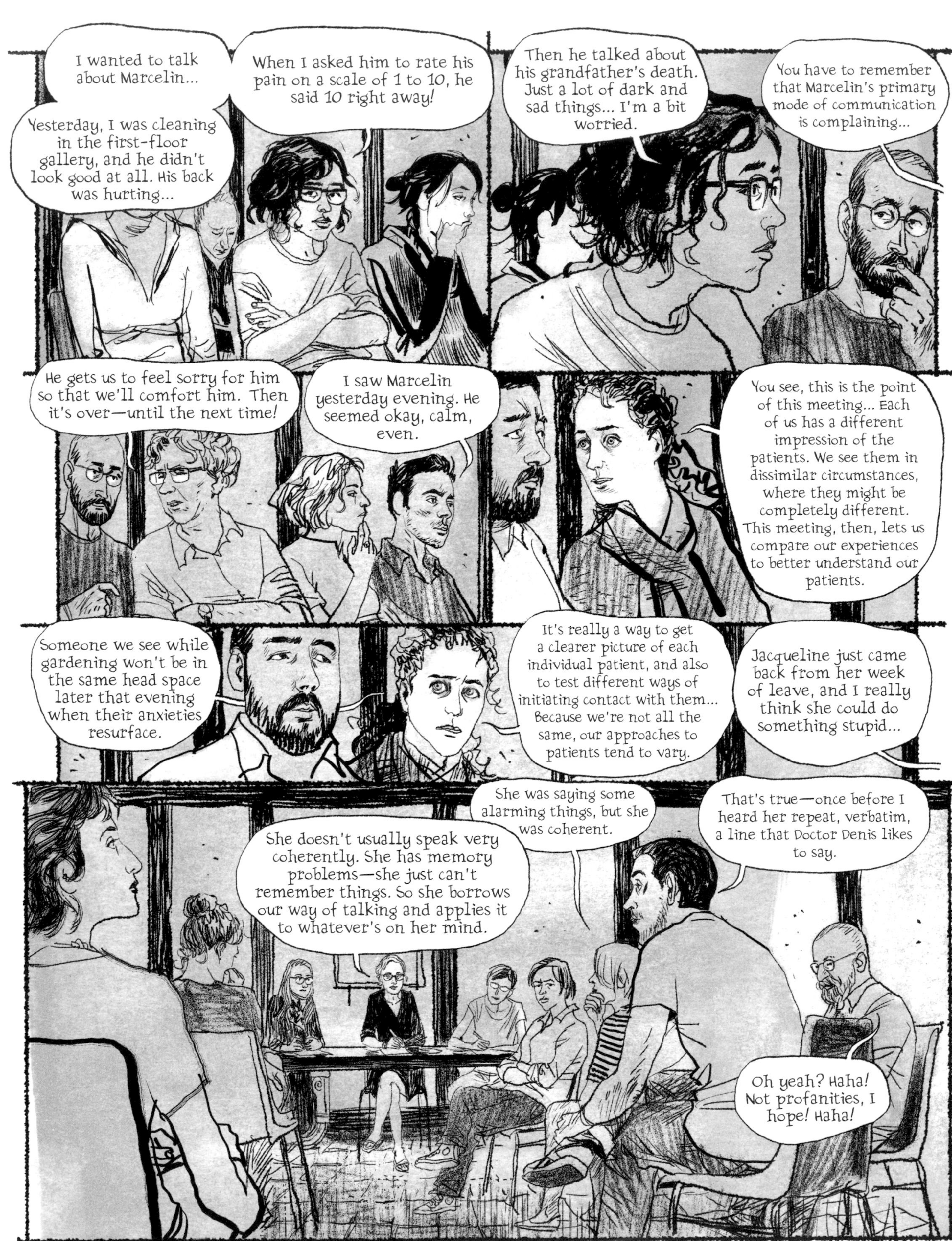
I wanted to talk about Marcelin...
Yesterday, I was cleaning in the first-floor gallery, and he didn't look good at all. His back was hurting...
When I asked him to rate his pain on a scale of 1 to 10, he said 10 right away!
Then he talked about his grandfather's death. Just a lot of dark and sad things... I'm a bit worried.
You have to remember that Marcelin's primary mode of communication is complaining...
He gets us to feel sorry for him so that we'll comfort him. Then it's over—until the next time!
I saw Marcelin yesterday evening. He seemed okay, calm, even.
You see, this is the point of this meeting... Each of us has a different impression of the patients. We see them in dissimilar circumstances, where they might be completely different. This meeting, then, lets us compare our experiences to better understand our patients.
Someone we see while gardening won't be in the same head space later that evening when their anxieties resurface.
It's really a way to get a clearer picture of each individual patient, and also to test different ways of initiating contact with them... Because we're not all the same, our approaches to patients tend to vary.
Jacqueline just came back from her week of leave, and I really think she could do something stupid...
She was saying some alarming things, but she was coherent.
She doesn't usually speak very coherently. She has memory problems—she just can't remember things. So she borrows our way of talking and applies it to whatever's on her mind.
That's true—once before I heard her repeat, verbatim, a line that Doctor Denis likes to say.
Oh yeah? Haha! Not profanities, I hope! Haha!

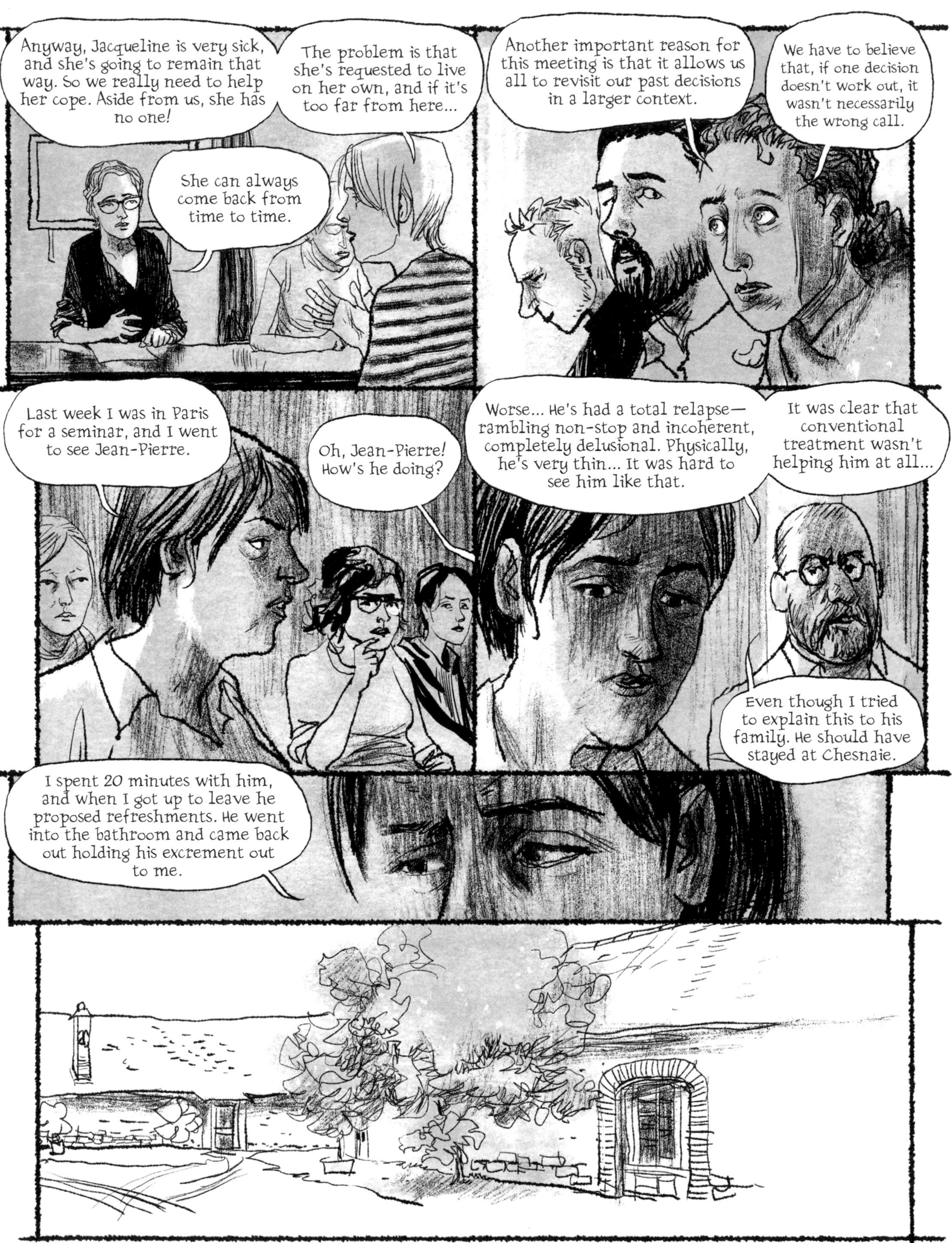
Anyway, Jacqueline is very sick, and she's going to remain that way. So we really need to help her cope. Aside from us, she has no one!
The problem is that she's requested to live on her own, and if it's too far from here...
She can always come back from time to time.
Another important reason for this meeting is that it allows us all to revisit our past decisions in a larger context.
We have to believe that, if one decision doesn't work out, it wasn't necessarily the wrong call.
Last week I was in Paris for a seminar, and I went to see Jean-Pierre.
Oh, Jean-Pierre! How's he doing?
Worse... He's had a total relapse— rambling non-stop and incoherent, completely delusional. Physically, he's very thin... It was hard to see him like that.
It was clear that conventional treatment wasn't helping him at all...
Even though I tried to explain this to his family. He should have stayed at Chesnaie.
I spent 20 minutes with him, and when I got up to leave he proposed refreshments. He went into the bathroom and came back out holding his excrement out to me.

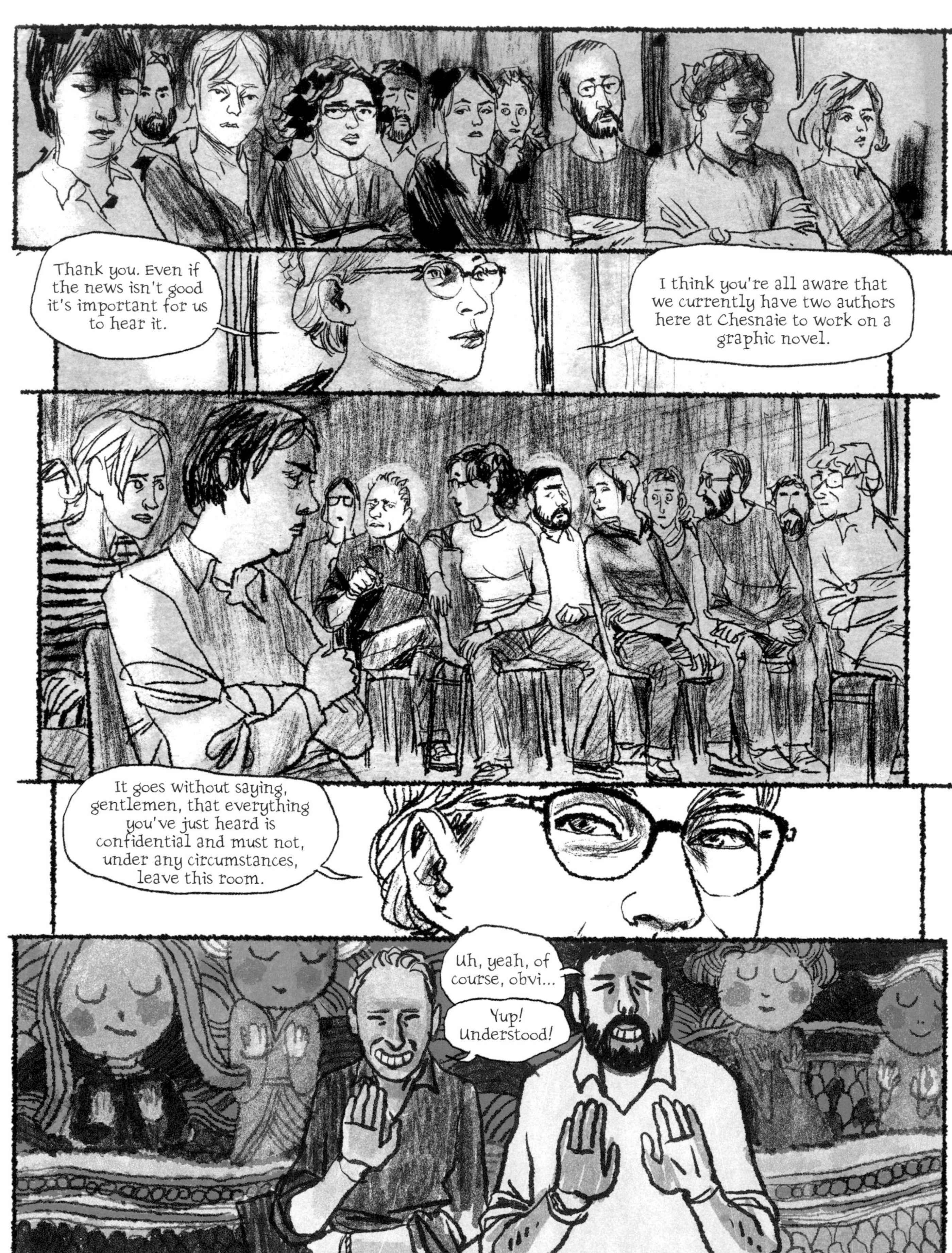
Thank you. Even if the news isn't good it's important for us to hear it.
I think you're all aware that we currently have two authors here at Chesnaie to work on a graphic novel.
It goes without saying, gentlemen, that everything you've just heard is confidential and must not, under any circumstances, leave this room.
Uh, yeah, of course, obvi...
Yup! Understood!

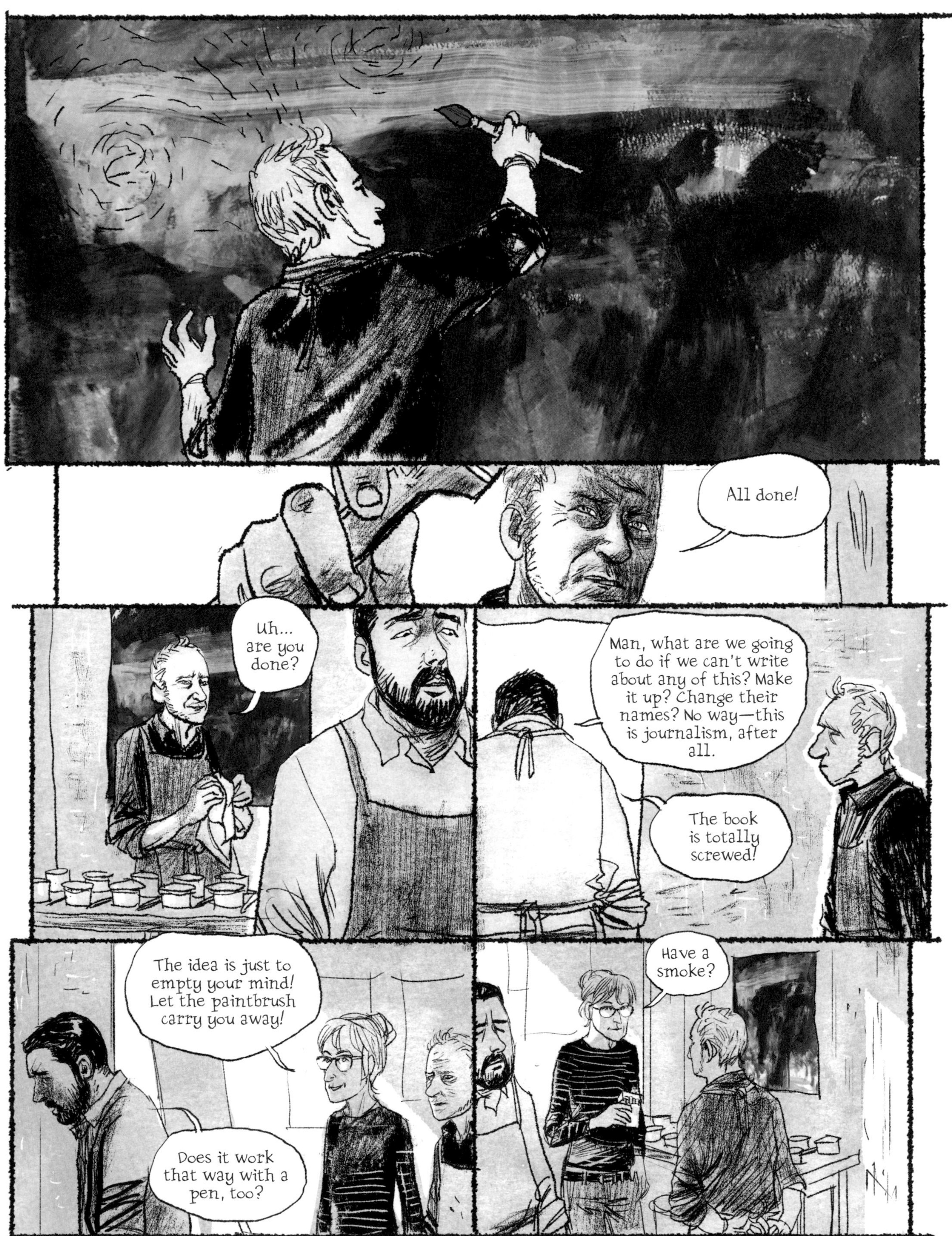
All done!
Uh... are you done?
Man, what are we going to do if we can't write about any of this? Make it up? Change their names? No way—this is journalism, after all.
The book is totally screwed!
The idea is just to empty your mind! Let the paintbrush carry you away!
Does it work that way with a pen, too?
Have a smoke?

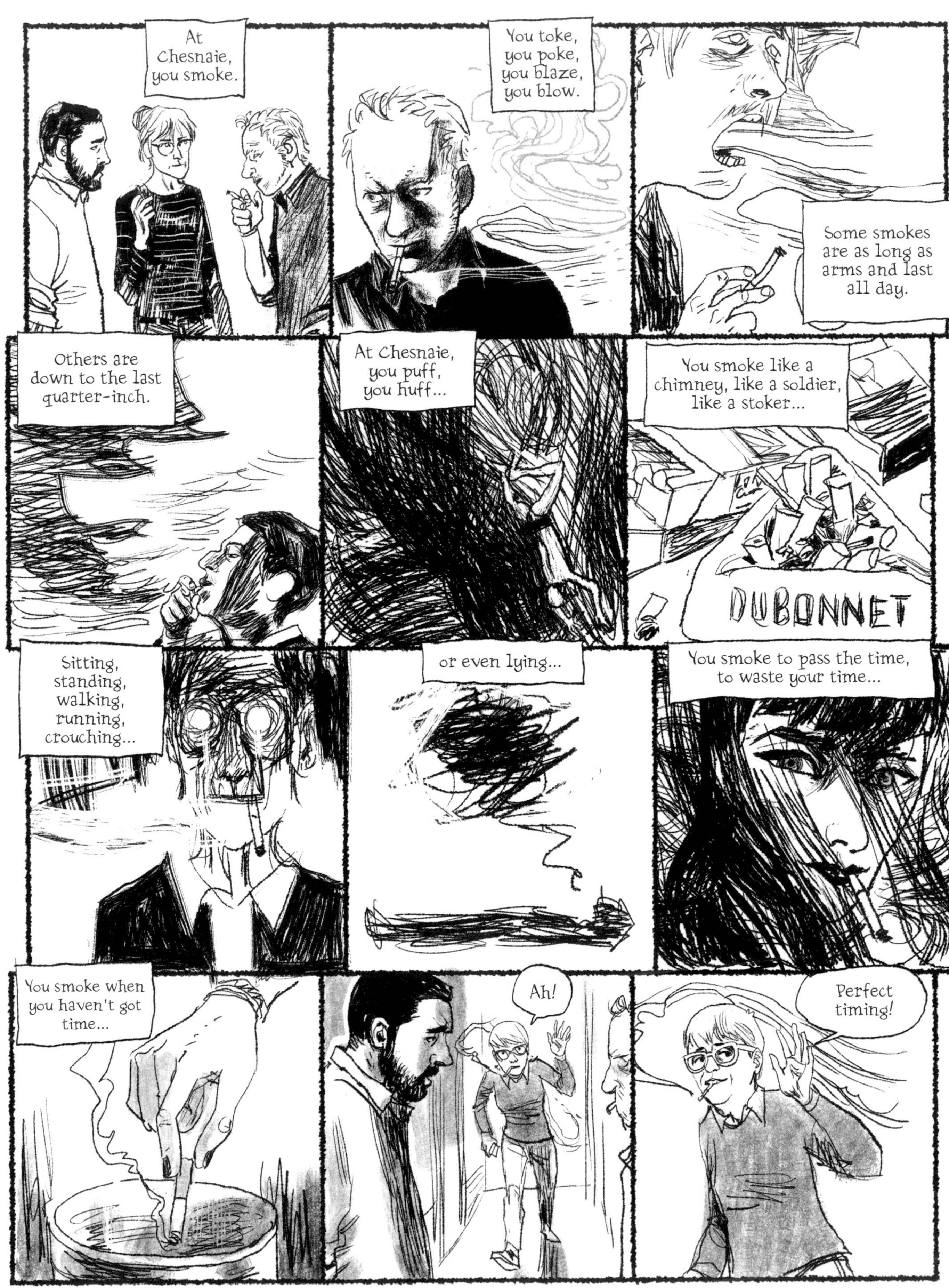
At Chesnaie, you smoke.
You toke, you poke, you blaze, you blow.
Some smokes are as long as arms and last all day.
Others are down to the last quarter-inch.
At Chesnaie, you puff, you huff...
You smoke like a chimney, like a soldier, like a stoker...
DUBONNET
Sitting, standing, walking, running, crouching...
or even lying...
You smoke to pass the time, to waste your time...
You smoke when you haven't got time...
Ah!
Perfect timing!

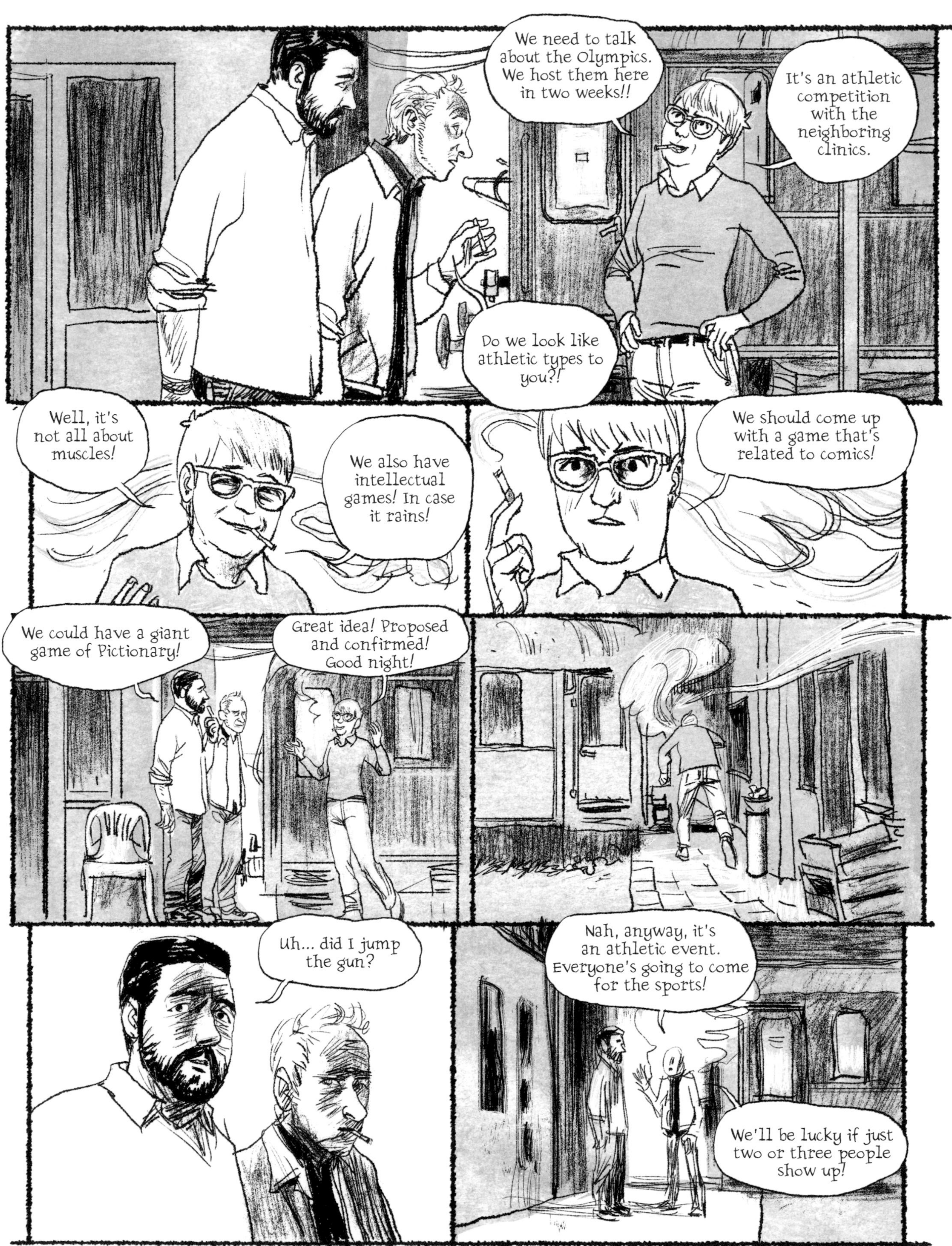
We need to talk about the Olympics. We host them here in two weeks!!
It's an athletic competition with the neighboring clinics.
Do we look like athletic types to you?!
Well, it's not all about muscles!
We also have intellectual games! In case it rains!
We should come up with a game that's related to comics!
We could have a giant game of Pictionary!
Great idea! Proposed and confirmed! Good night!
Uh... did I jump the gun?
Nah, anyway, it's an athletic event. Everyone's going to come for the sports!
We'll be lucky if just two or three people show up!

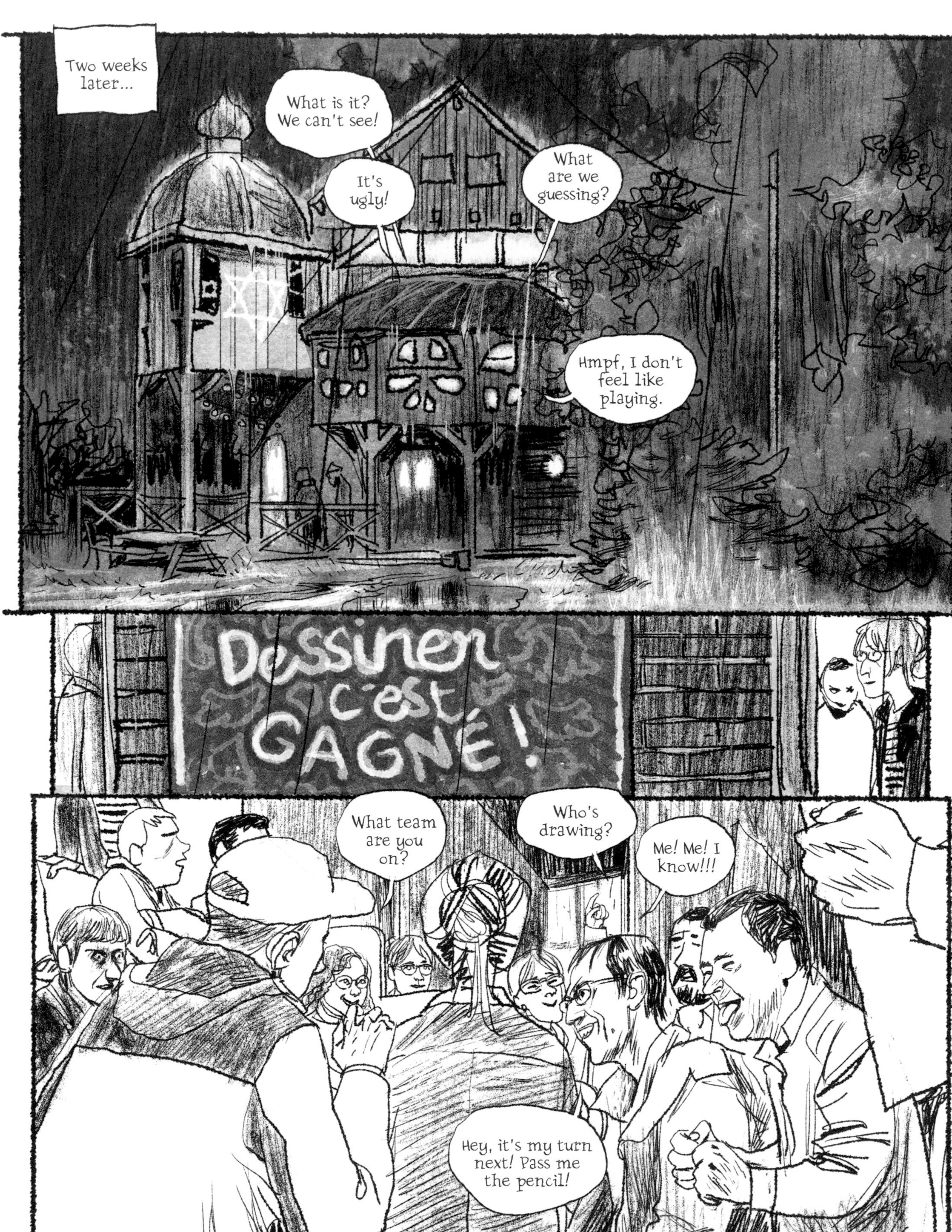
Two weeks later...
What is it? We can't see!
It's ugly!
What are we guessing?
Hmpf, I don't feel like playing.
Dessiner c'est GAGNÉ!
What team are you on?
Who's drawing?
Me! Me! I know!!!
Hey, it's my turn next! Pass me the pencil!

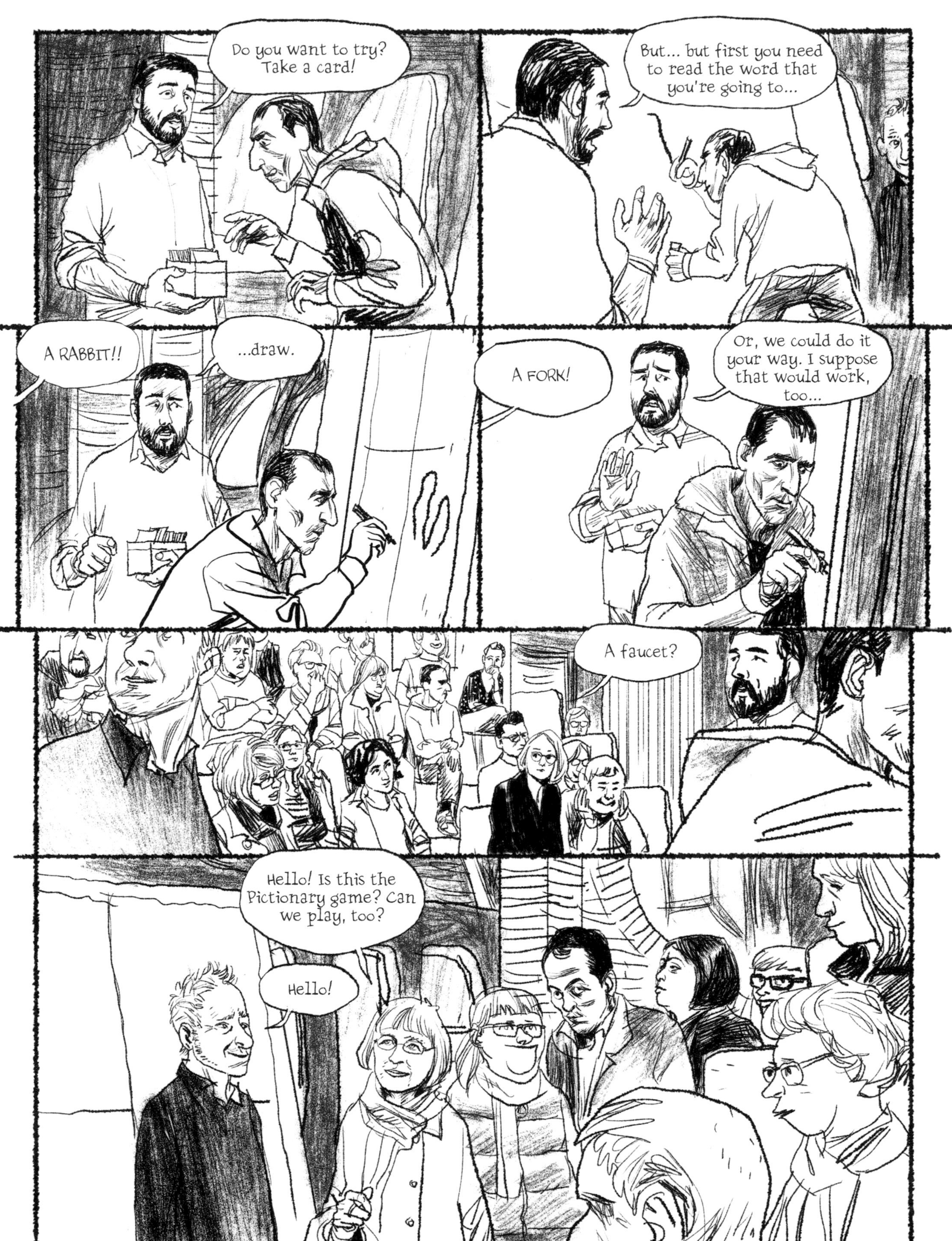
Do you want to try? Take a card!
But... but first you need to read the word that you're going to...
A RABBIT!!
...draw.
A FORK!
Or, we could do it your way. I suppose that would work, too...
A faucet?
Hello! Is this the Pictionary game? Can we play, too?
Hello!

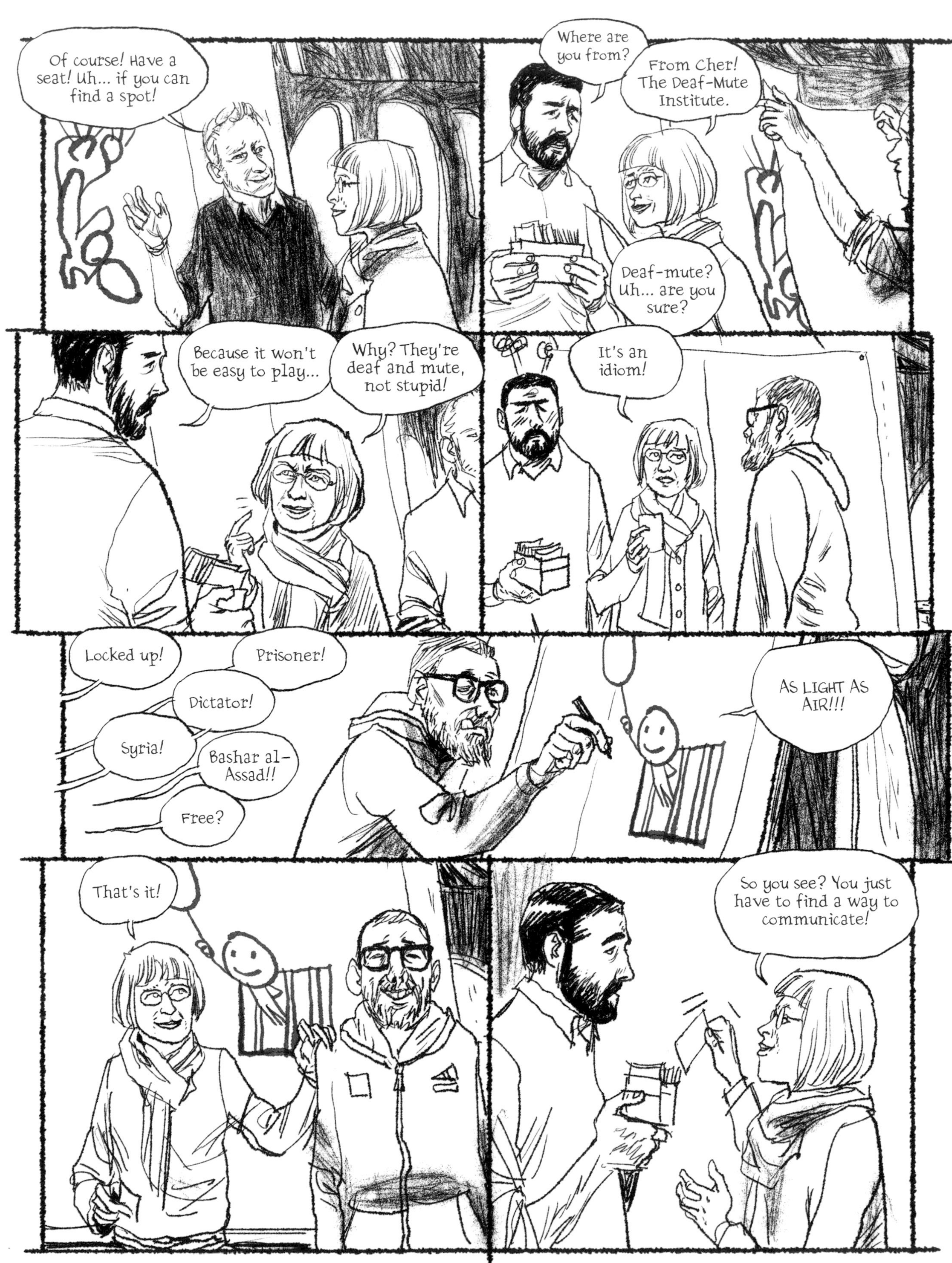
Of course! Have a seat! Uh... if you can find a spot!
Where are you from?
From Cher! The Deaf-Mute Institute.
Deaf-mute? Uh... are you sure?
Because it won't be easy to play...
Why? They're deaf and mute, not stupid!
It's an idiom!
Locked up!
Prisoner!
Dictator!
Syria!
Bashar al-Assad!!
Free?
AS LIGHT AS AIR!!!
That's it!
So you see? You just have to find a way to communicate!

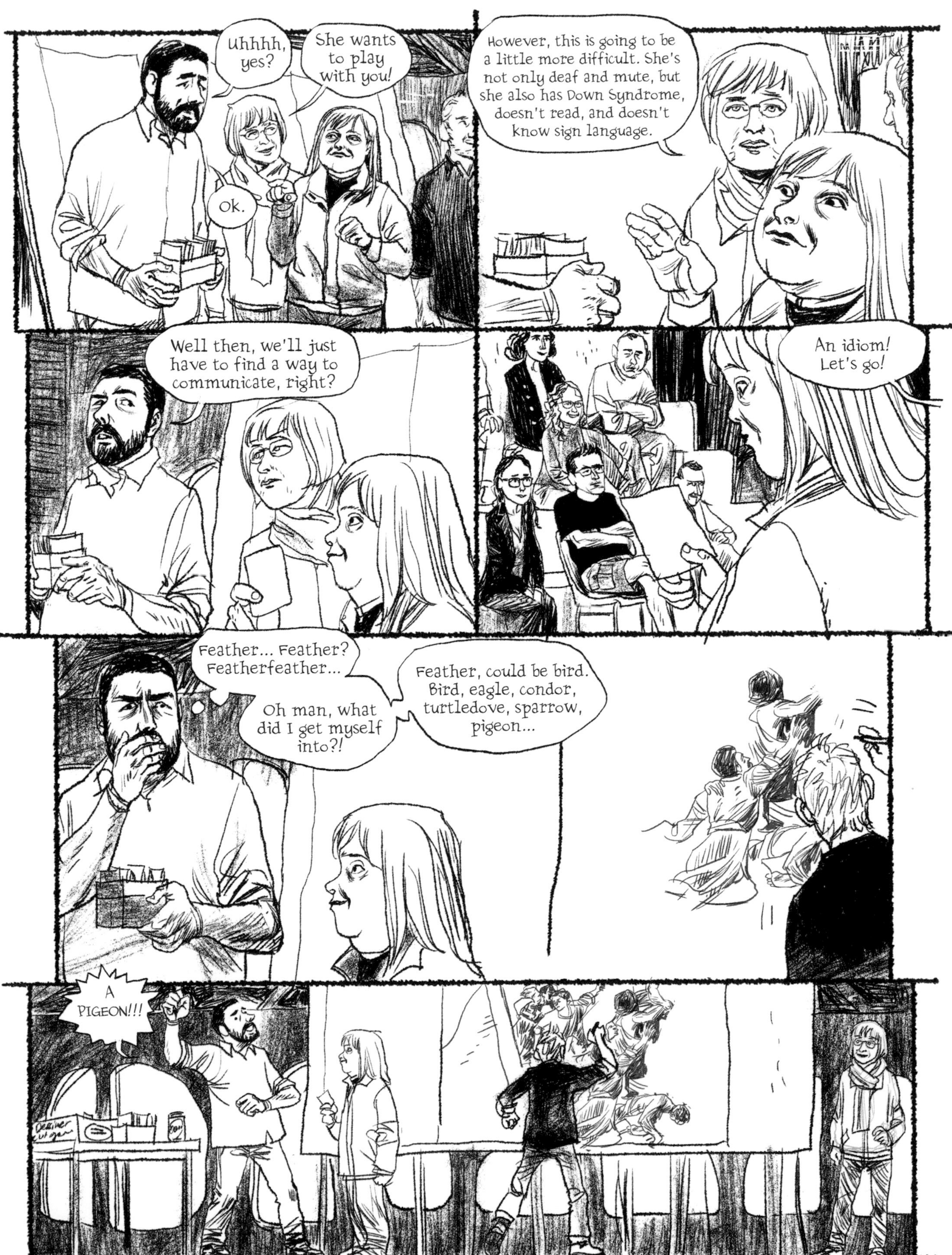
Uhhhh, yes?
She wants to play with you!
Ok.
However, this is going to be a little more difficult. She's not only deaf and mute, but she also has Down Syndrome, doesn't read, and doesn't know sign language.
Well then, we'll just have to find a way to communicate, right?
An idiom! Let's go!
Feather... Feather? Featherfeather...
Oh man, what did I get myself into?!
Feather, could be bird. Bird, eagle, condor, turtledove, sparrow, pigeon...
A PIGEON!!!

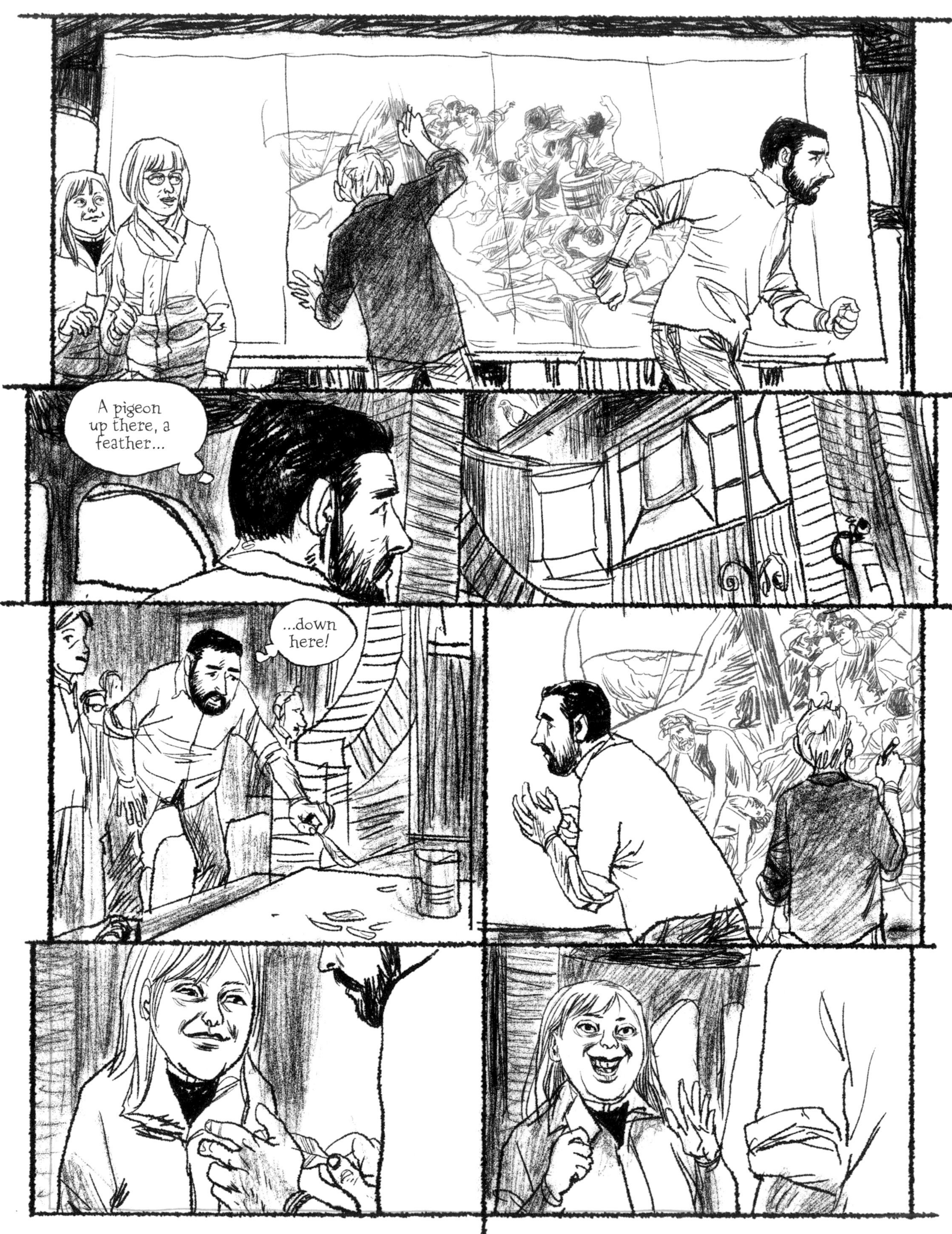
A pigeon up there, a feather...
...down here!

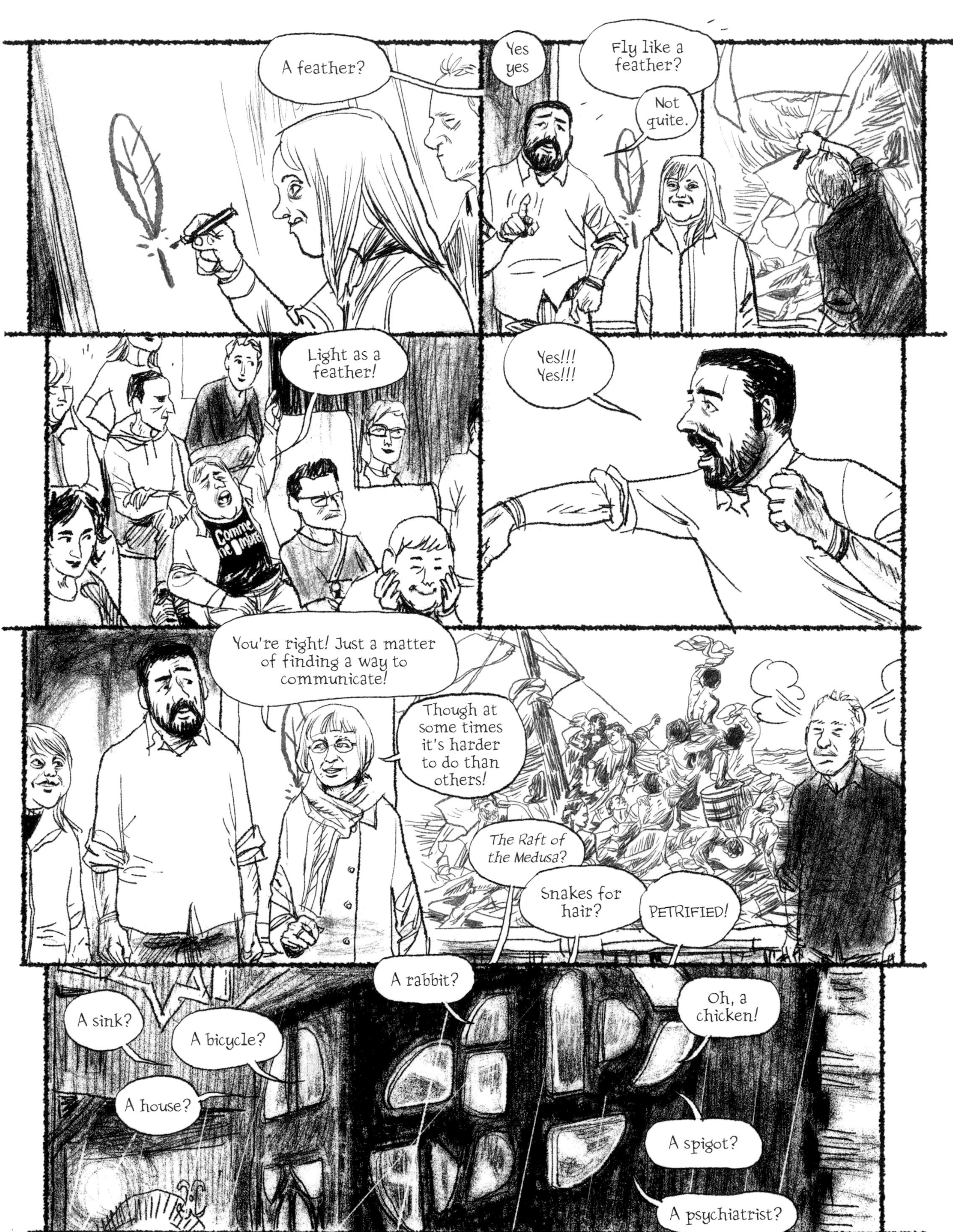
A feather?
Yes yes
Fly like a feather?
Not quite.
Light as a feather!
Yes!!! Yes!!!
You're right! Just a matter of finding a way to communicate!
Though at some times it's harder to do than others!
The Raft of the Medusa?
Snakes for hair?
PETRIFIED!
A sink?
A bicycle?
A house?
A rabbit?
Oh, a chicken!
A spigot?
A psychiatrist?

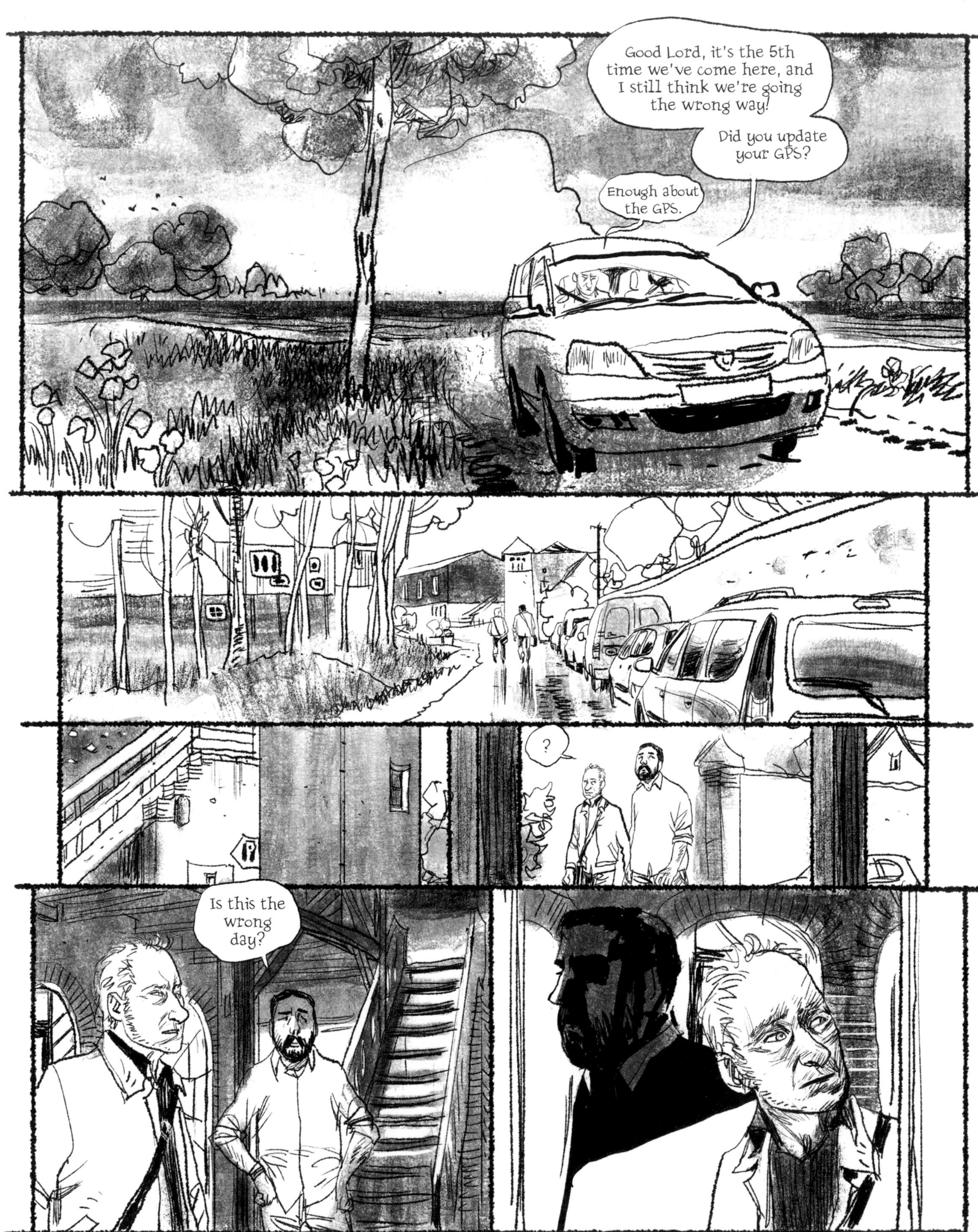

Good Lord, it's the 5th time we've come here, and I still think we're going the wrong way!
Did you update your GPS?
Enough about the GPS.
?
Is this the wrong day?

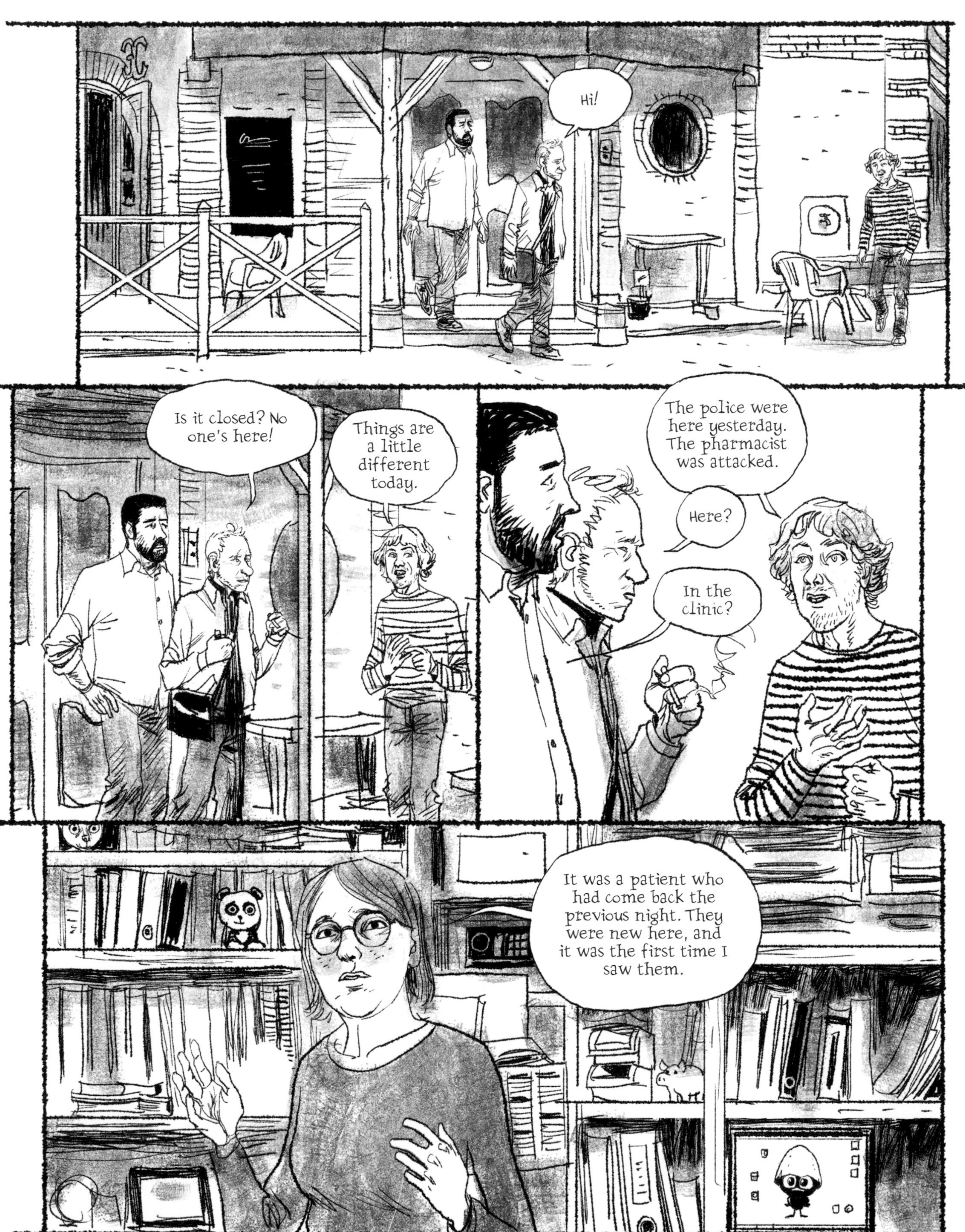
Hi!
Is it closed? No one's here!
Things are a little different today.
The police were here yesterday. The pharmacist was attacked.
Here?
In the clinic?
It was a patient who had come back the previous night. They were new here, and it was the first time I saw them.

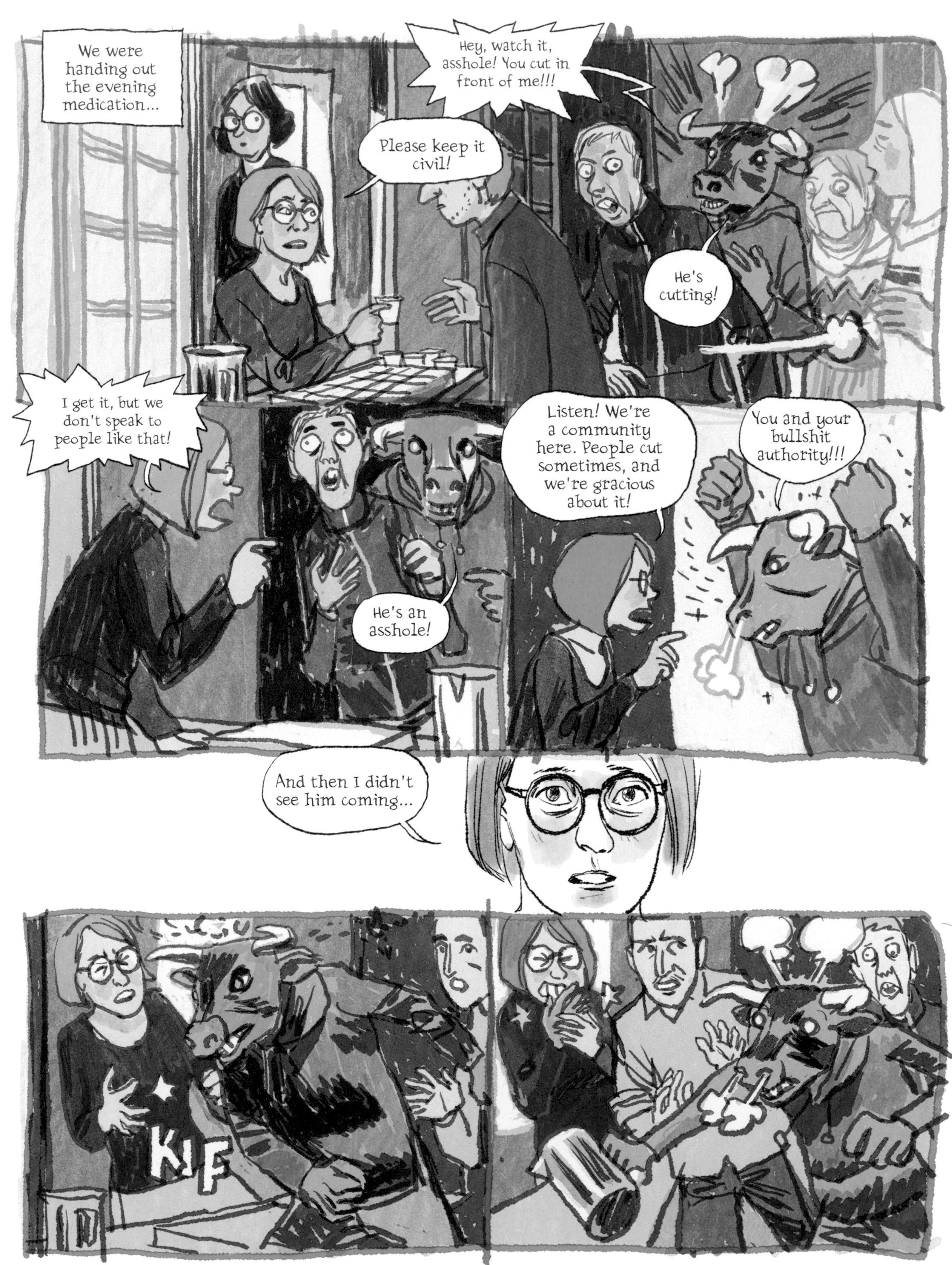
We were handing out the evening medication...
Please keep it civil!
Hey, watch it, asshole! You cut in front of me!!!
He's cutting!
I get it, but we don't speak to people like that!
He's an asshole!
Listen! We're a community here. People cut sometimes, and we're gracious about it!
You and your bullshit authority!!!
And then I didn't see him coming...
KIF

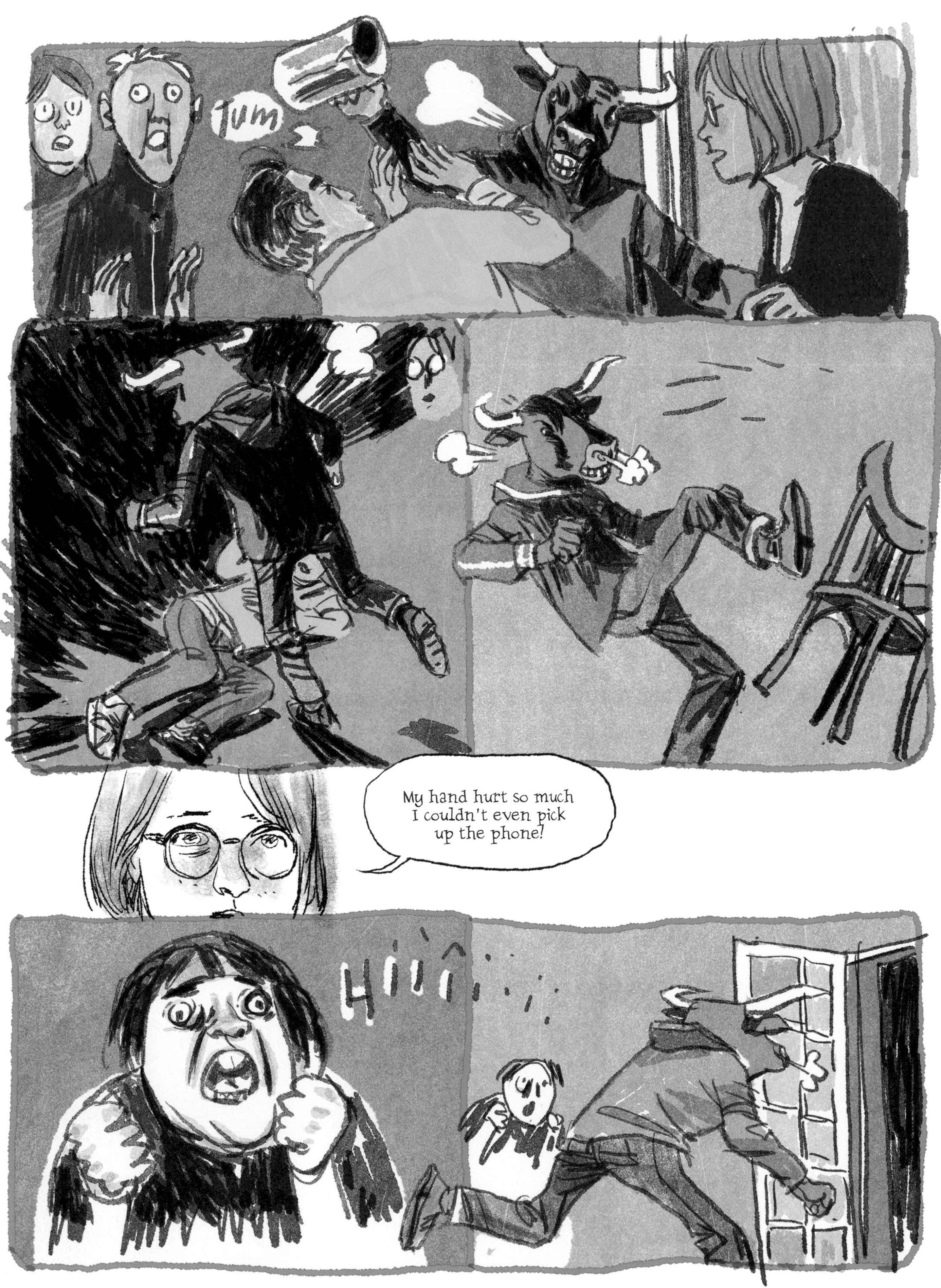
TUM
My hand hurt so much I couldn't even pick up the phone!
HIII

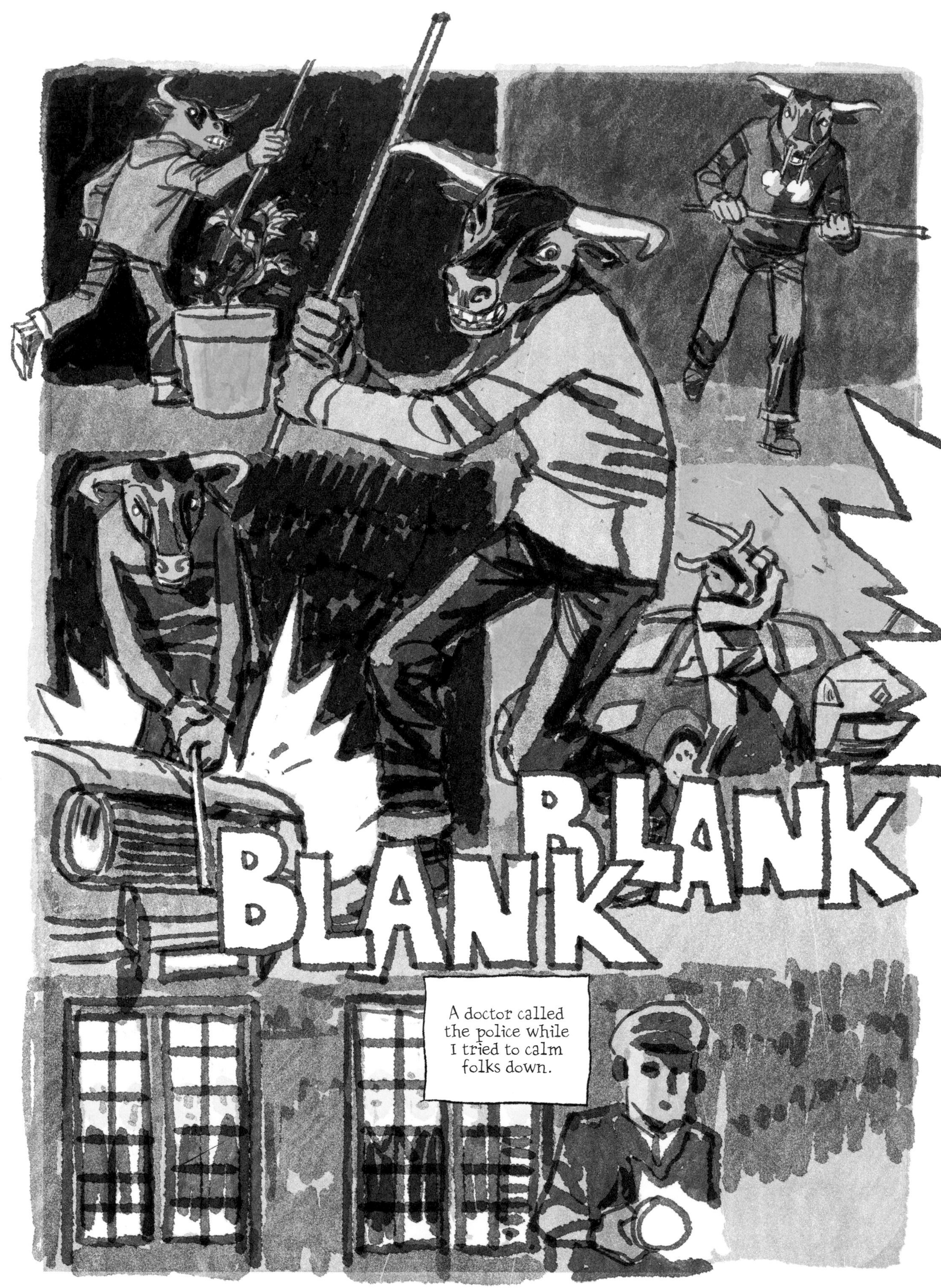
BLANK
BLANK
A doctor called the police while I tried to calm folks down.

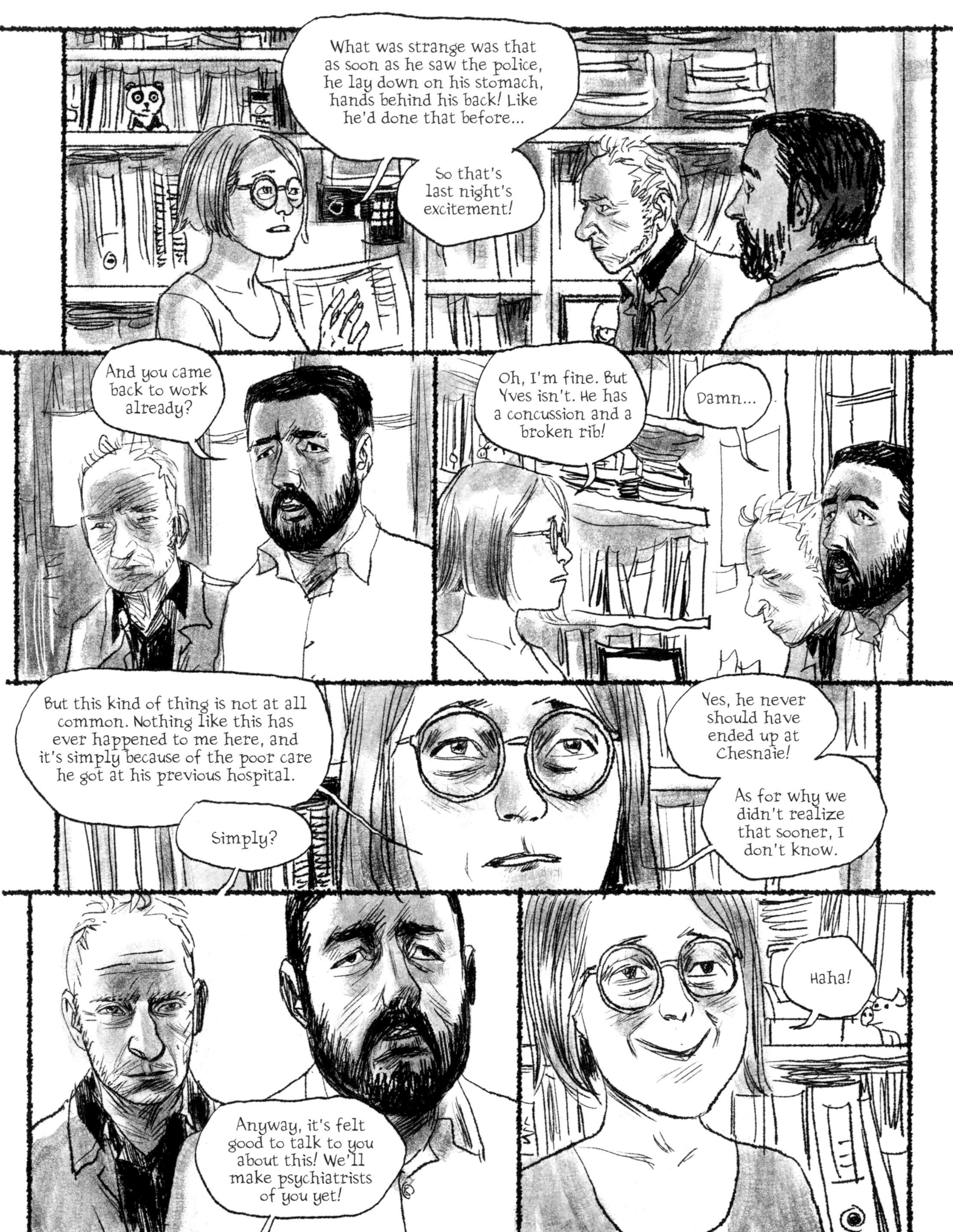
What was strange was that as soon as he saw the police, he lay down on his stomach, hands behind his back! Like he'd done that before...
So that's last night's excitement!
And you came back to work already?
Oh, I'm fine. But Yves isn't. He has a concussion and a broken rib!
Damn...
But this kind of thing is not at all common. Nothing like this has ever happened to me here, and it's simply because of the poor care he got at his previous hospital.
Simply?
Yes, he never should have ended up at Chesnaie!
As for why we didn't realize that sooner, I don't know.
Anyway, it's felt good to talk to you about this! We'll make psychiatrists of you yet!
Haha!

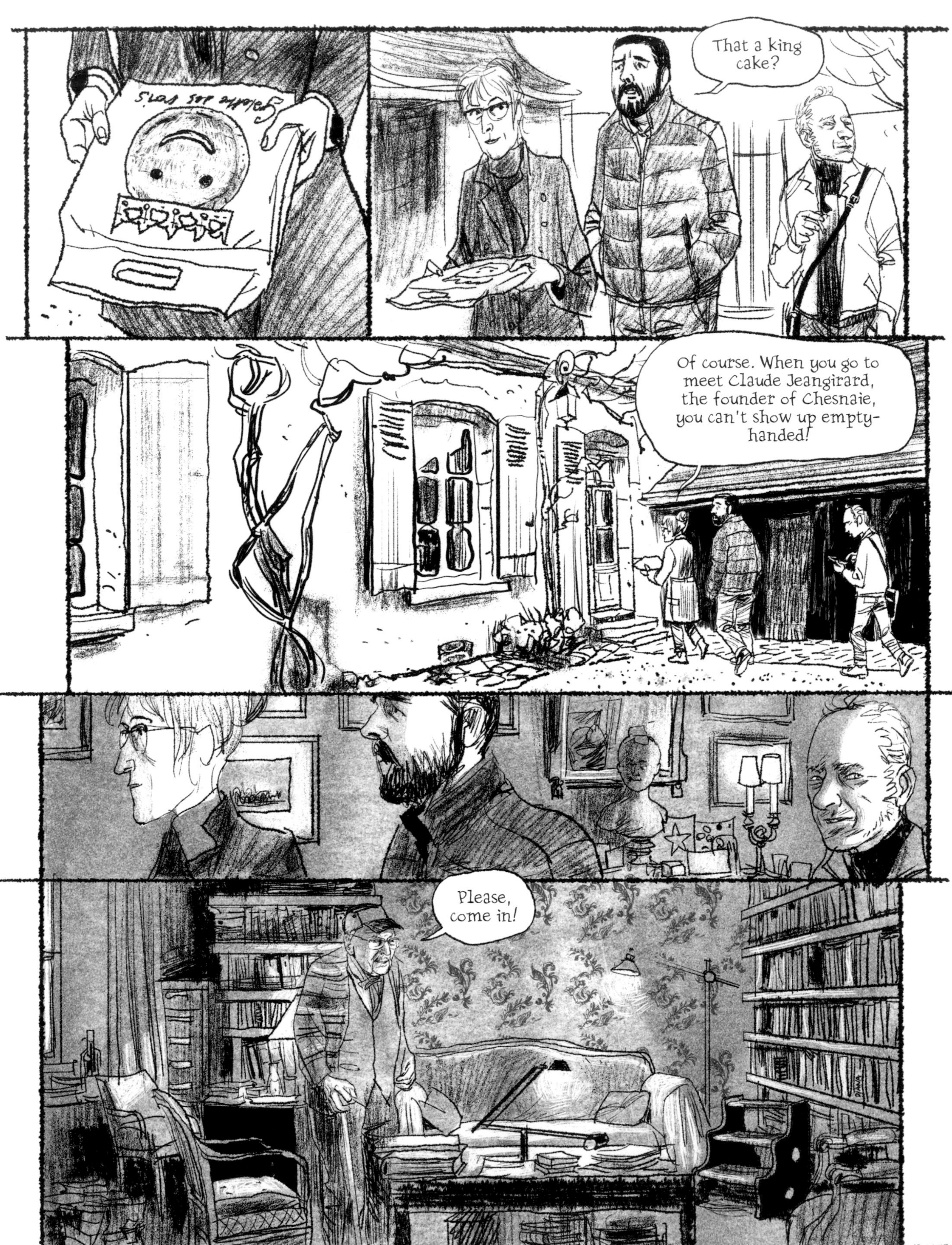
That a king cake?
Of course. When you go to meet Claude Jeangirard, the founder of Chesnaie, you can't show up empty-handed!
Please, come in!

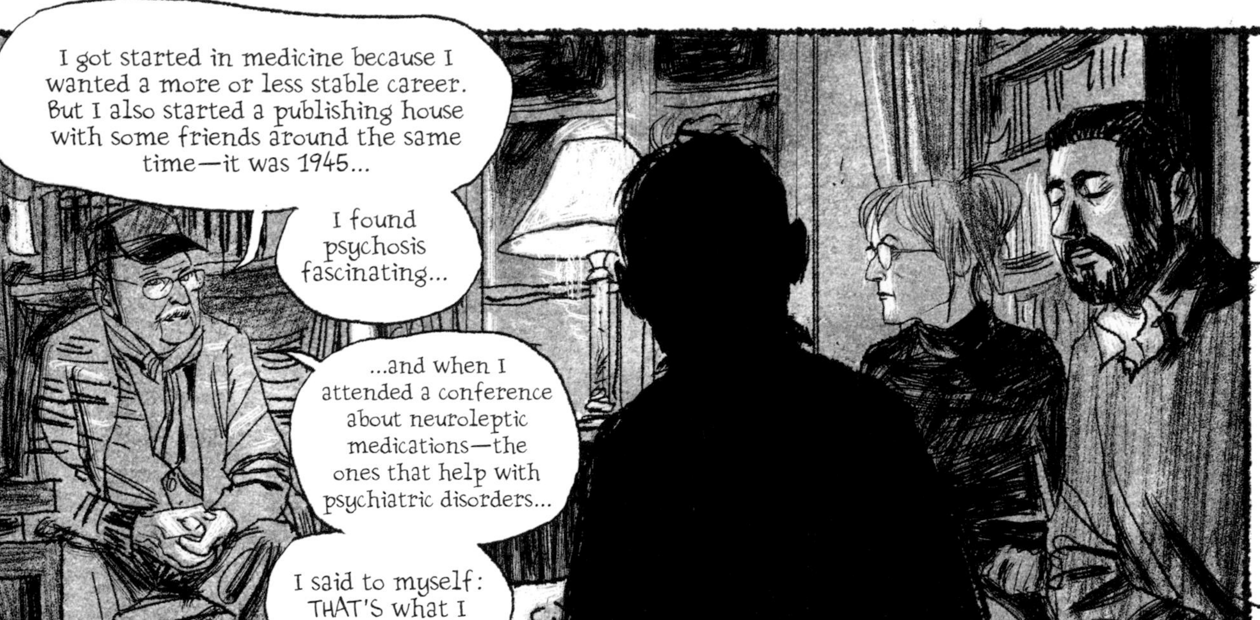

I got started in medicine because I wanted a more or less stable career. But I also started a publishing house with some friends around the same time—it was 1945...
I found psychosis fascinating...
...and when I attended a conference about neuroleptic medications—the ones that help with psychiatric disorders...
I said to myself: THAT'S what I want to do!

So I took up practice in Sainte-Anne, replacing another colleague, and that brought me into this fringe medical community, which included Parisian intellectuals and my friends from the publishing world... It goes without saying that I spent a lot of time at the theater!

Intellectuals, poets and writers, surrealists, Antonin Artaud, they were all interested in psychosis.

People at first thought psychosis was just gibberish, but we knew there was something there. Something to learn about, understand, and build on—and we tried hard to avoid misunderstanding!

It's like a door opened for us.

You know, psychosis is a type of mental illness that wasn't recognized until we had liberty, equality, and fraternity...

The revolutionaries of 1789 thought that people with mental illness—usually either ignored or criminalized—weren't receiving the medical care they needed.

In 1838, as an effect of the "Age of Enlightenment," the National Assembly decided to recognize the insane and find a way to care for them—that is, to commit them to insane asylums.

There was one asylum for each of the 95 French departments, an expensive project run by a new kind of doctor called "Alienists," who were both the directors of these psychiatric hospitals and the scientists.

In Blois, for example, the psychiatric hospital and the insane asylum took up an entire neighborhood!

Later, the war provided an opportunity to discharge the Blois asylees. After the exodus of 1940, they were found wandering about the countryside. They were admitted to nearby hospitals, and in the Blois asylum they set up an administrative center and three high schools! So you can imagine how huge this place was!

So, back to psychosis. Where was I?

Psychosis essentially shows up in a 15-year-old boy or girl who resents their parents, cuts school, sleeps all day, smokes cigarettes, and exhibits increasingly bizarre behavior. As their relationship with their mother becomes more and more intimate and regressive, they develop recurring schizophrenic delusions...

Well, that's the classic pattern for chronic delusion, and it builds on a number of ideas developed as far back as the 19th century, including omnipotence, megalomania, and other signs of psychotic rupture.

Someone with psychosis is non-productive by definition. They can't contribute to society in the way others do. Of course they're interested in what's going on in the world, but their outlook tends to be highly critical and delusional, and that's not at all constructive...

That's why even the well-meaning and generous among us have been inclined to confine them and feed them but ask nothing of them in return...

And then there's Chesnaie. The delusional tendencies of patients here have evolved in different ways... Sometimes when a patient's serious delusions stop, they're able to become friends, to a certain degree, with those of us who aren't in treatment.

But psychosis is still psychosis, even if the people suffering from it manage to grow in ways that expand their social and emotional lives.

After a certain amount of time, they can take part in the kinds of associative structures that allow for productivity.

If we could extend Chesnaie's reach beyond Chesnaie, we could help a large number of psychotics who are unique members of society but are really no stranger than artists or other types!

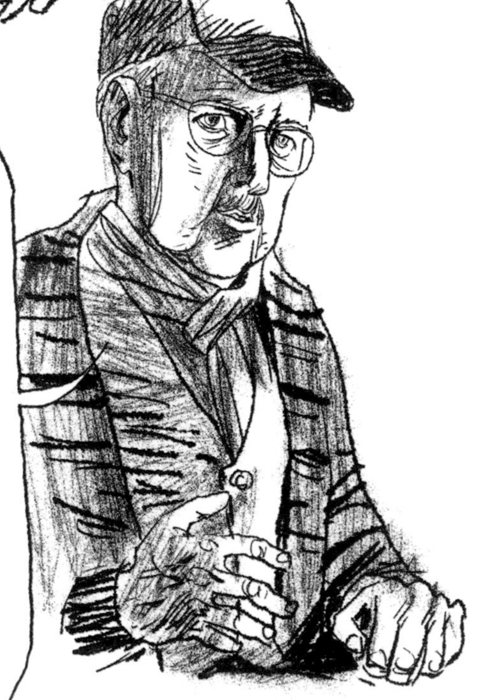

Now, obviously, the government doesn't support what I'm telling you here. They favor behaviorism, the one-size-fits-all approach where you treat symptoms with large doses of medications.

The patient with psychosis, when he's treated well in the institutions, has a close relationship with a caregiver. Psychosis is binary. You can recognize a psychotic as follows. You're speaking with someone in the street when, all of a sudden, a person springs out right in front of you, and without pausing, launches into a conversation. Of course they don't recognize that you're already busy talking to someone else. That's psychosis. It's no more complicated than that. So, if you're aware of that, there's no point in scolding the person by saying, "You're bothering me, you're impolite," etc. It never occurs to you to say that.

In an institution, the first caregiver a patient latches onto, and who can continue the relationship through the ups and downs of life, will be a very important source of support for the patient...

Unfortunately, that's not the current approach, because today one caregiver can easily replace another. But that's wrong! We all have patients that we've become rather attached to...

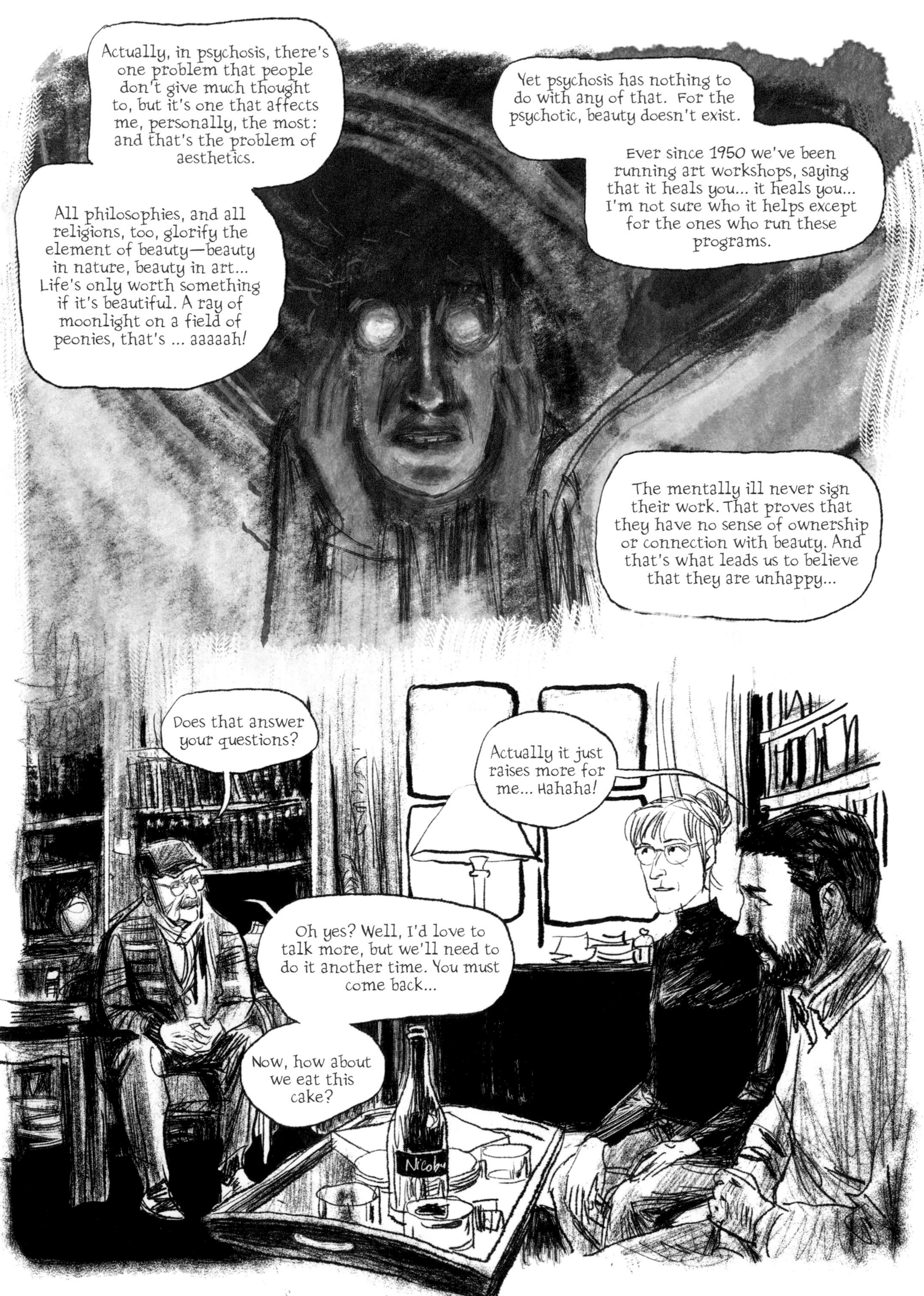
Actually, in psychosis, there's one problem that people don't give much thought to, but it's one that affects me, personally, the most: and that's the problem of aesthetics.
All philosophies, and all religions, too, glorify the element of beauty—beauty in nature, beauty in art... Life's only worth something if it's beautiful. A ray of moonlight on a field of peonies, that's ... aaaaah!
Yet psychosis has nothing to do with any of that. For the psychotic, beauty doesn't exist.
Ever since 1950 we've been running art workshops, saying that it heals you... it heals you... I'm not sure who it helps except for the ones who run these programs.
The mentally ill never sign their work. That proves that they have no sense of ownership or connection with beauty. And that's what leads us to believe that they are unhappy...
Does that answer your questions?
Actually it just raises more for me... Hahaha!
Oh yes? Well, I'd love to talk more, but we'll need to do it another time. You must come back...
Now, how about we eat this cake?
Nicobu

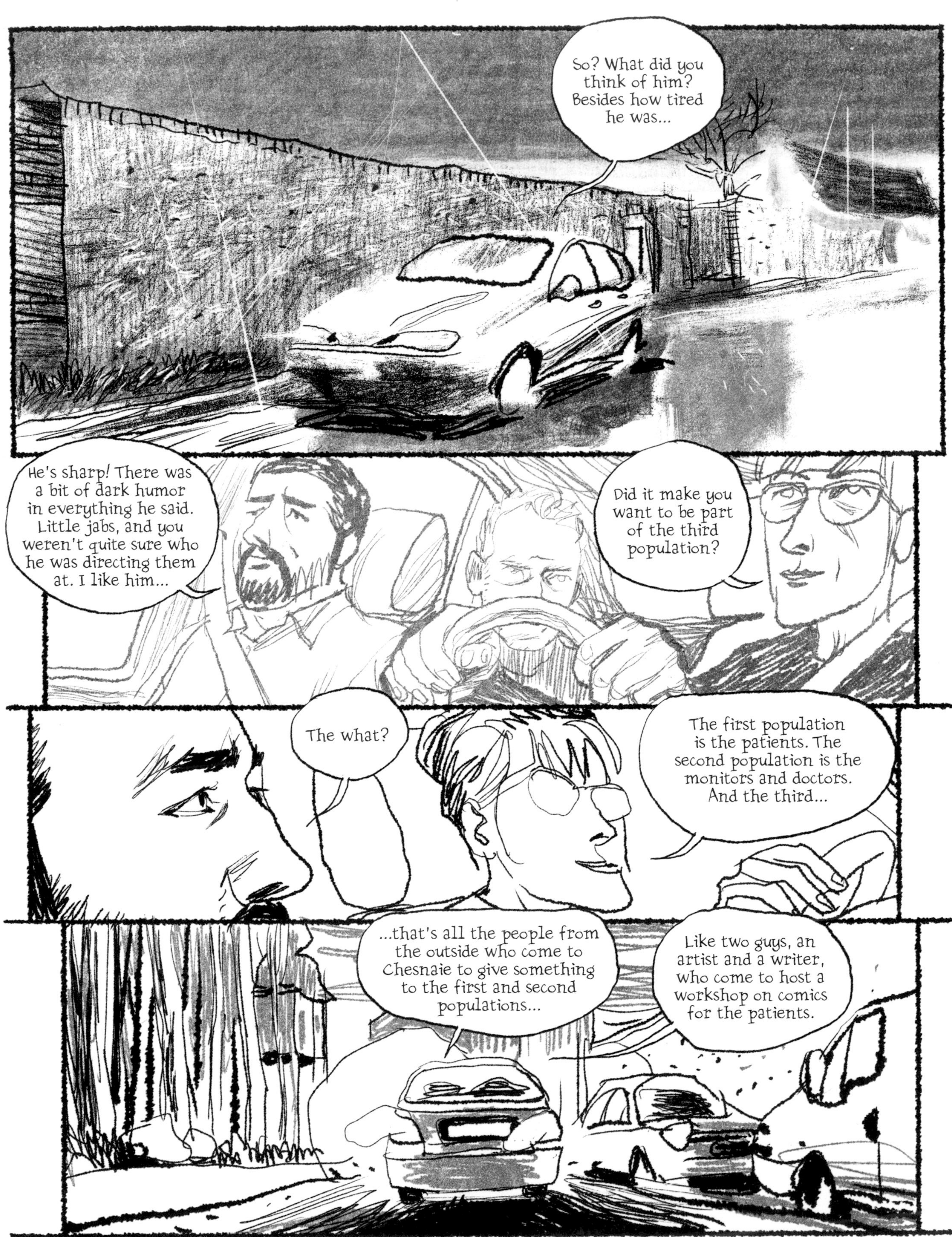
So? What did you think of him? Besides how tired he was...
He's sharp! There was a bit of dark humor in everything he said. Little jabs, and you weren't quite sure who he was directing them at. I like him...
Did it make you want to be part of the third population?
The what?
The first population is the patients. The second population is the monitors and doctors. And the third...
...that's all the people from the outside who come to Chesnaie to give something to the first and second populations...
Like two guys, an artist and a writer, who come to host a workshop on comics for the patients.

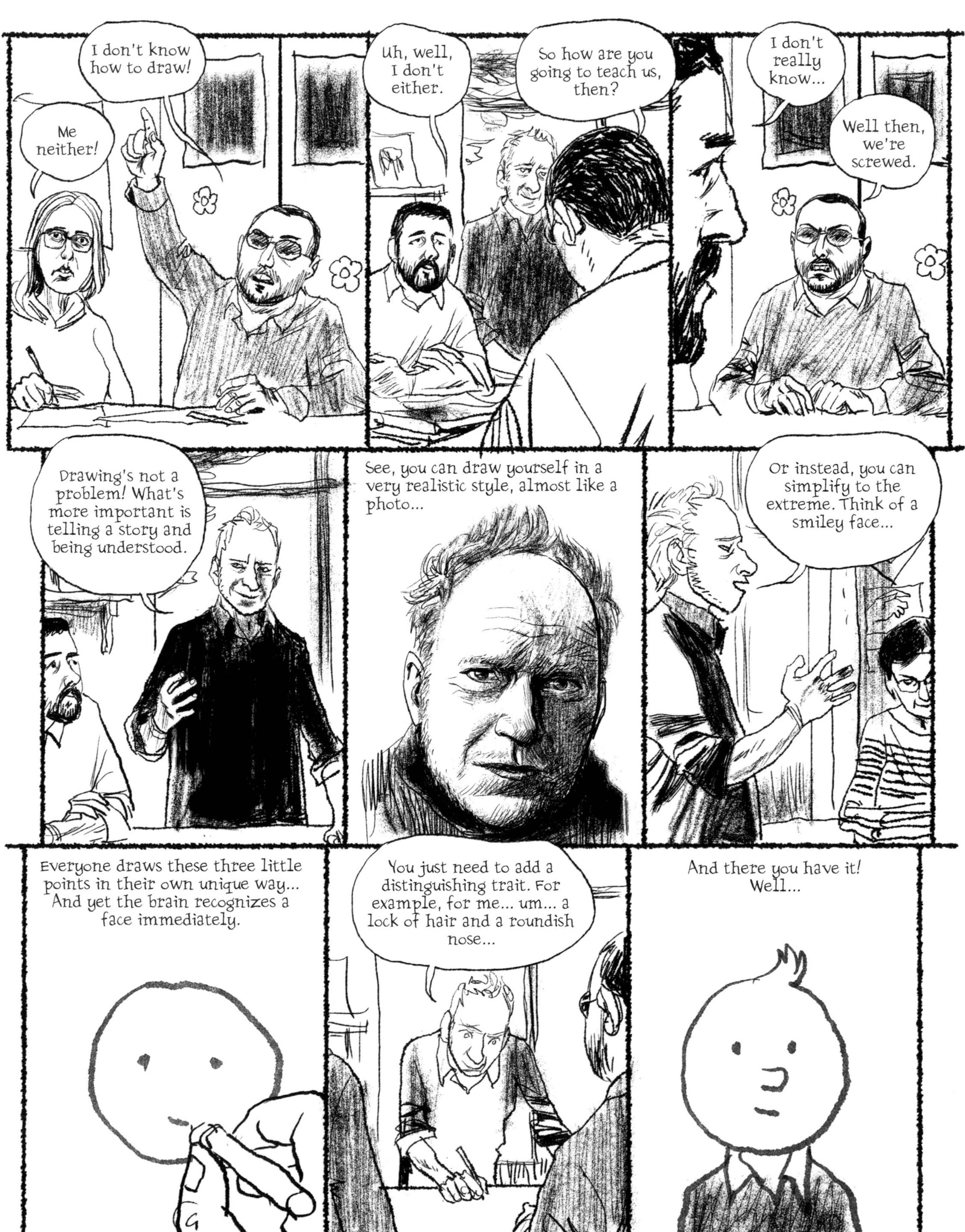

Me neither!
I don't know how to draw!
Uh, well, I don't either.
So how are you going to teach us, then?
I don't really know...
Well then, we're screwed.
Drawing's not a problem! What's more important is telling a story and being understood.
See, you can draw yourself in a very realistic style, almost like a photo...
Or instead, you can simplify to the extreme. Think of a smiley face...
Everyone draws these three little points in their own unique way... And yet the brain recognizes a face immediately.
You just need to add a distinguishing trait. For example, for me... um... a lock of hair and a roundish nose...
And there you have it! Well...

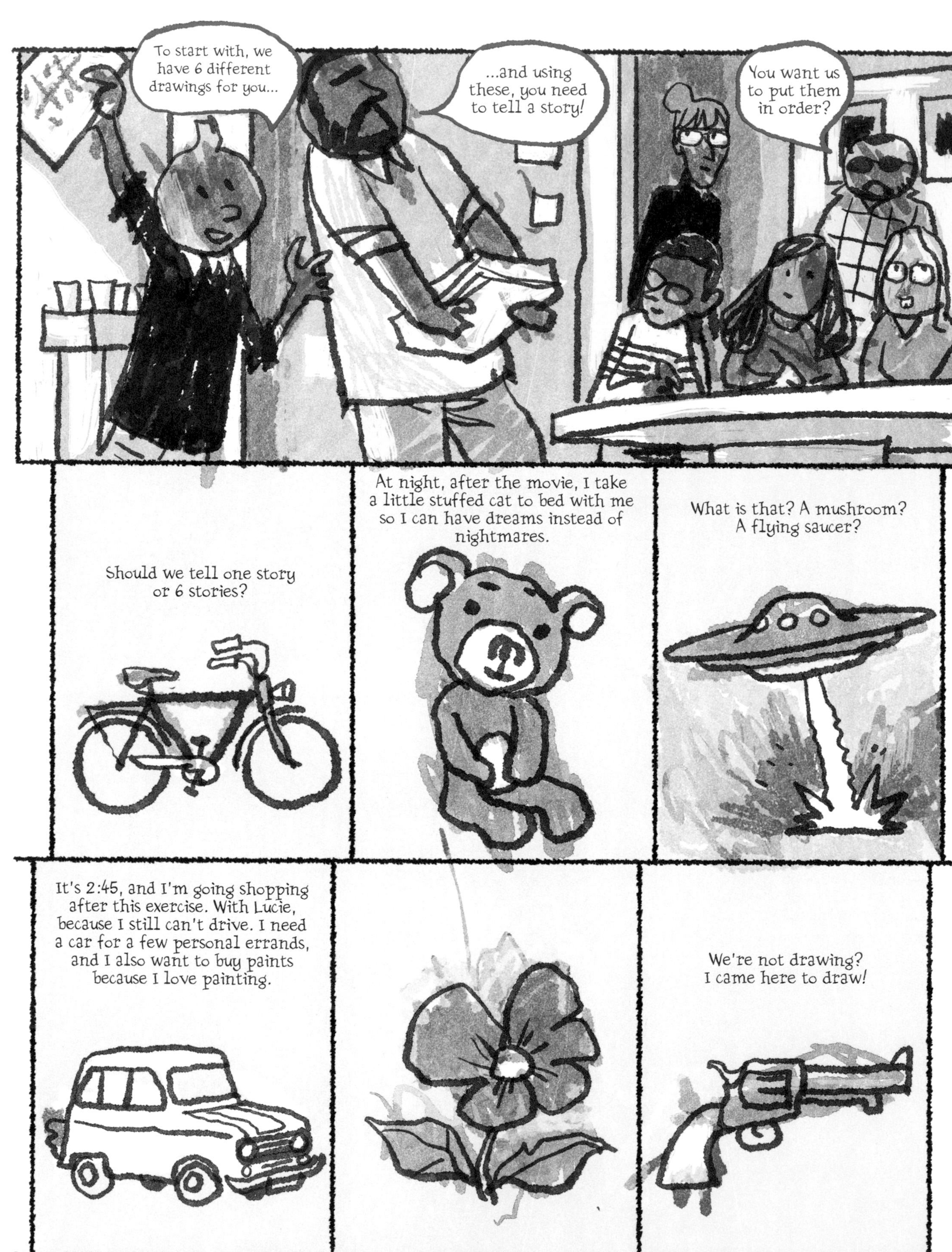
To start with, we have 6 different drawings for you...
...and using these, you need to tell a story!
You want us to put them in order?
Should we tell one story or 6 stories?
At night, after the movie, I take a little stuffed cat to bed with me so I can have dreams instead of nightmares.
What is that? A mushroom? A flying saucer?
It's 2:45, and I'm going shopping after this exercise. With Lucie, because I still can't drive. I need a car for a few personal errands, and I also want to buy paints because I love painting.
We're not drawing? I came here to draw!

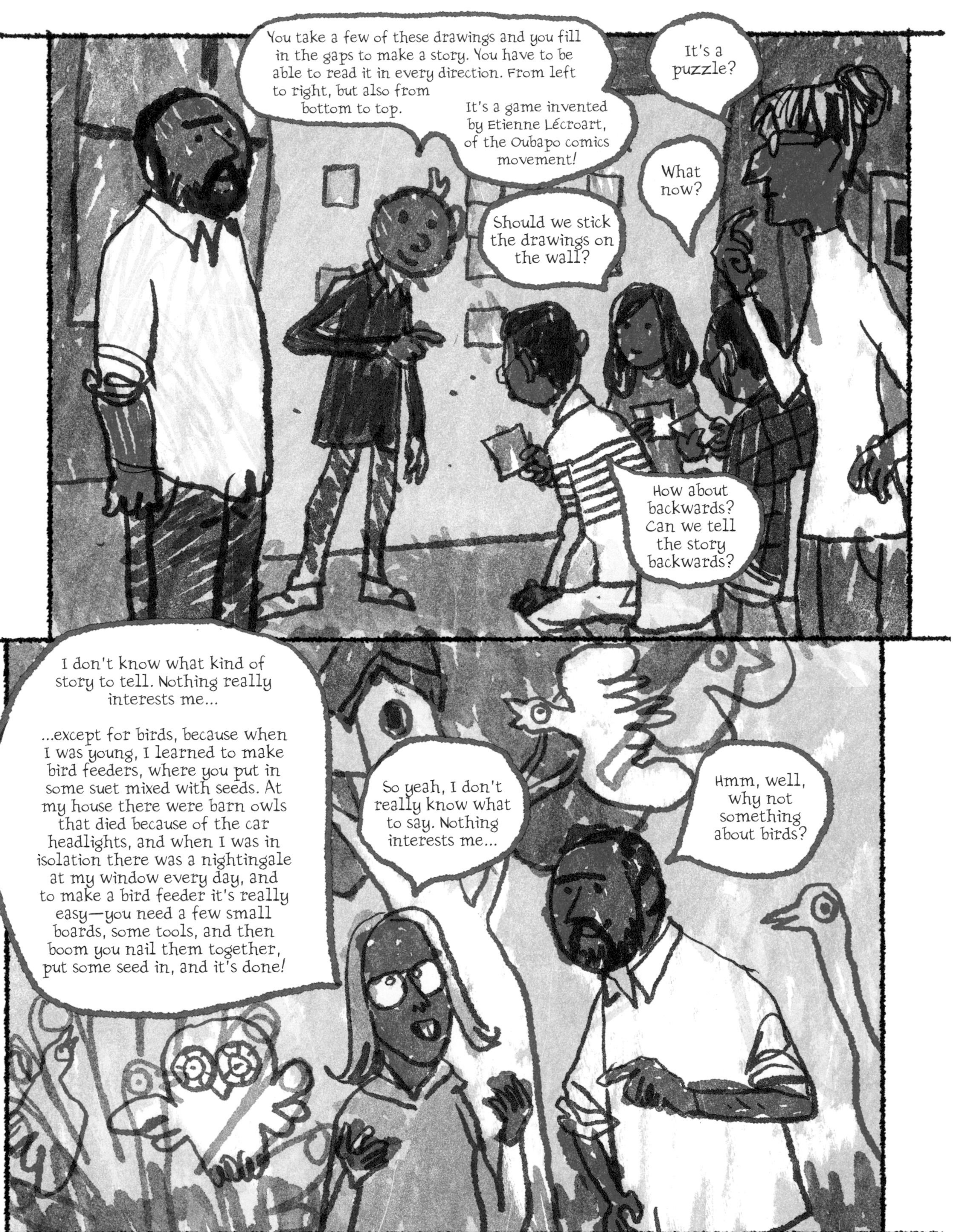
You take a few of these drawings and you fill in the gaps to make a story. You have to be able to read it in every direction. From left to right, but also from bottom to top.
It's a game invented by Etienne Lécroart, of the Oubapo comics movement!
It's a puzzle?
What now?
Should we stick the drawings on the wall?
How about backwards? Can we tell the story backwards?
I don't know what kind of story to tell. Nothing really interests me...
...except for birds, because when I was young, I learned to make bird feeders, where you put in some suet mixed with seeds. At my house there were barn owls that died because of the car headlights, and when I was in isolation there was a nightingale at my window every day, and to make a bird feeder it's really easy—you need a few small boards, some tools, and then boom you nail them together, put some seed in, and it's done!
So yeah, I don't really know what to say. Nothing interests me...
Hmm, well, why not something about birds?

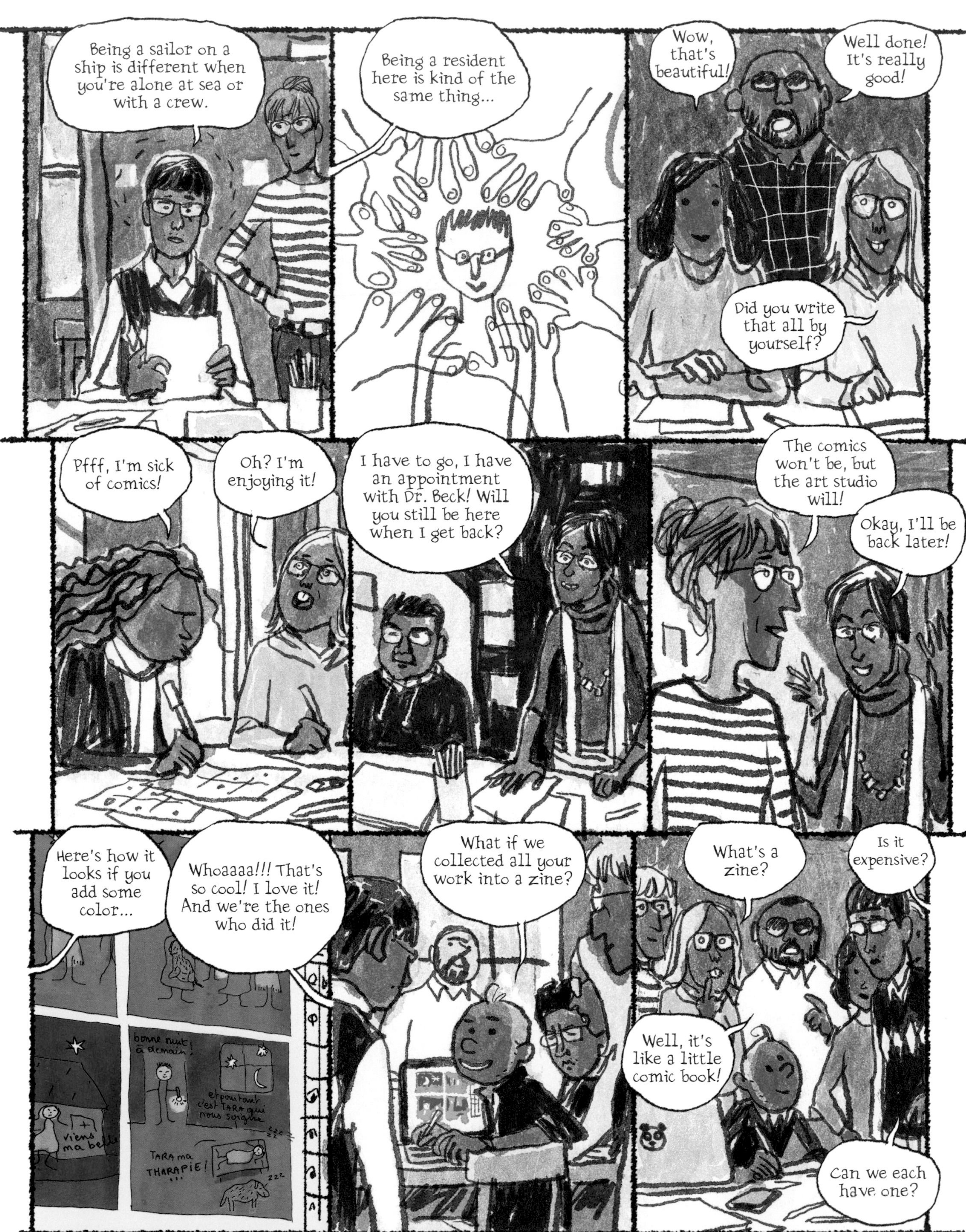

Being a sailor on a ship is different when you're alone at sea or with a crew.
Being a resident here is kind of the same thing...
Wow, that's beautiful!
Well done! It's really good!
Did you write that all by yourself?
Pfff, I'm sick of comics!
Oh? I'm enjoying it!
I have to go, I have an appointment with Dr. Beck! Will you still be here when I get back?
The comics won't be, but the art studio will!
Okay, I'll be back later!
Here's how it looks if you add some color...
Whoaaaa!!! That's so cool! I love it! And we're the ones who did it!
bonne nuit à demain!
et pourtant c'est TARA qui nous soigne
TARA ma THARAPIE!
What if we collected all your work into a zine?
What's a zine?
Is it expensive?
Well, it's like a little comic book!
Can we each have one?

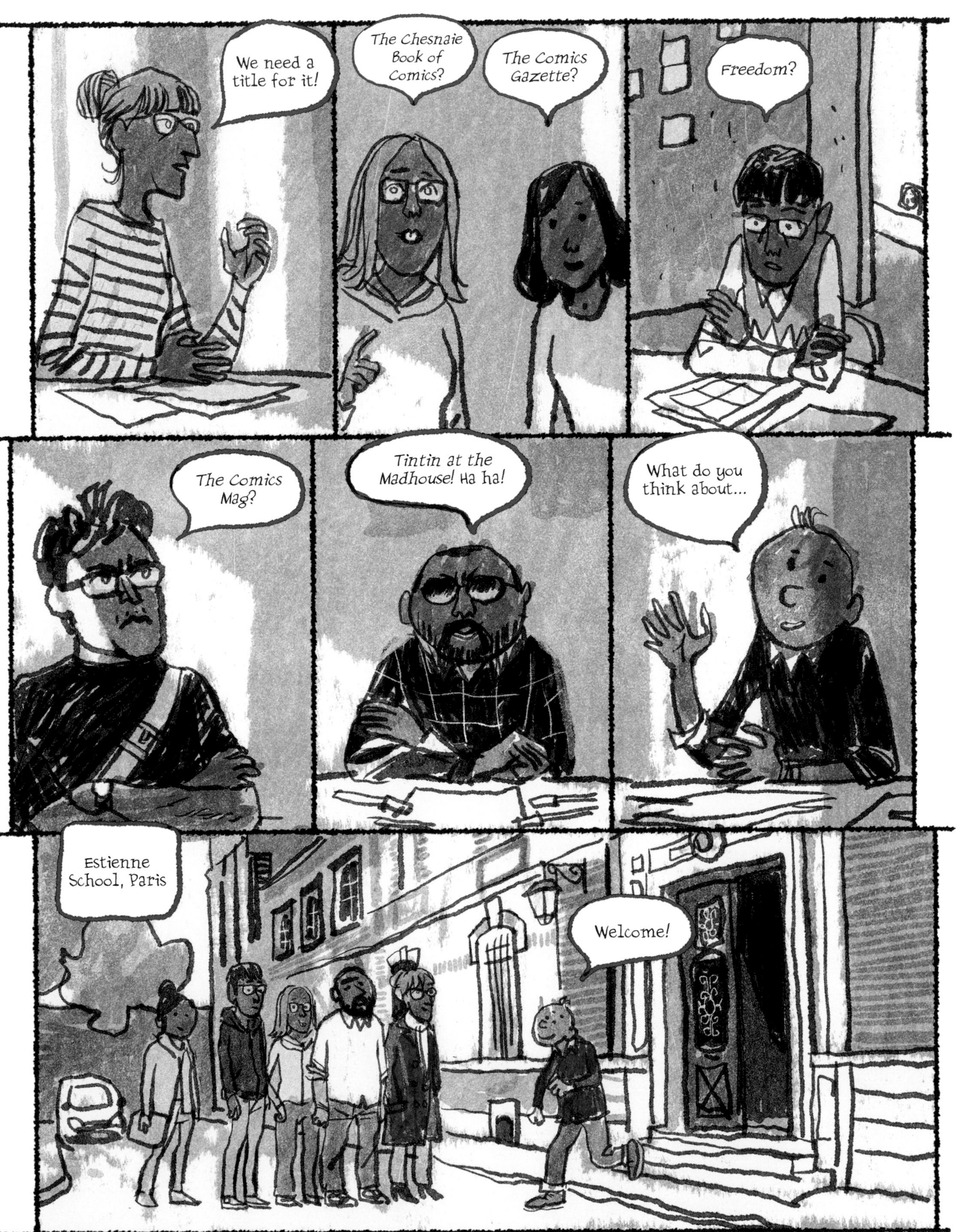
We need a title for it!
The Chesnaie Book of Comics?
The Comics Gazette?
Freedom?
The Comics Mag?
Tintin at the Madhouse! Ha ha!
What do you think about...
Estienne School, Paris
Welcome!

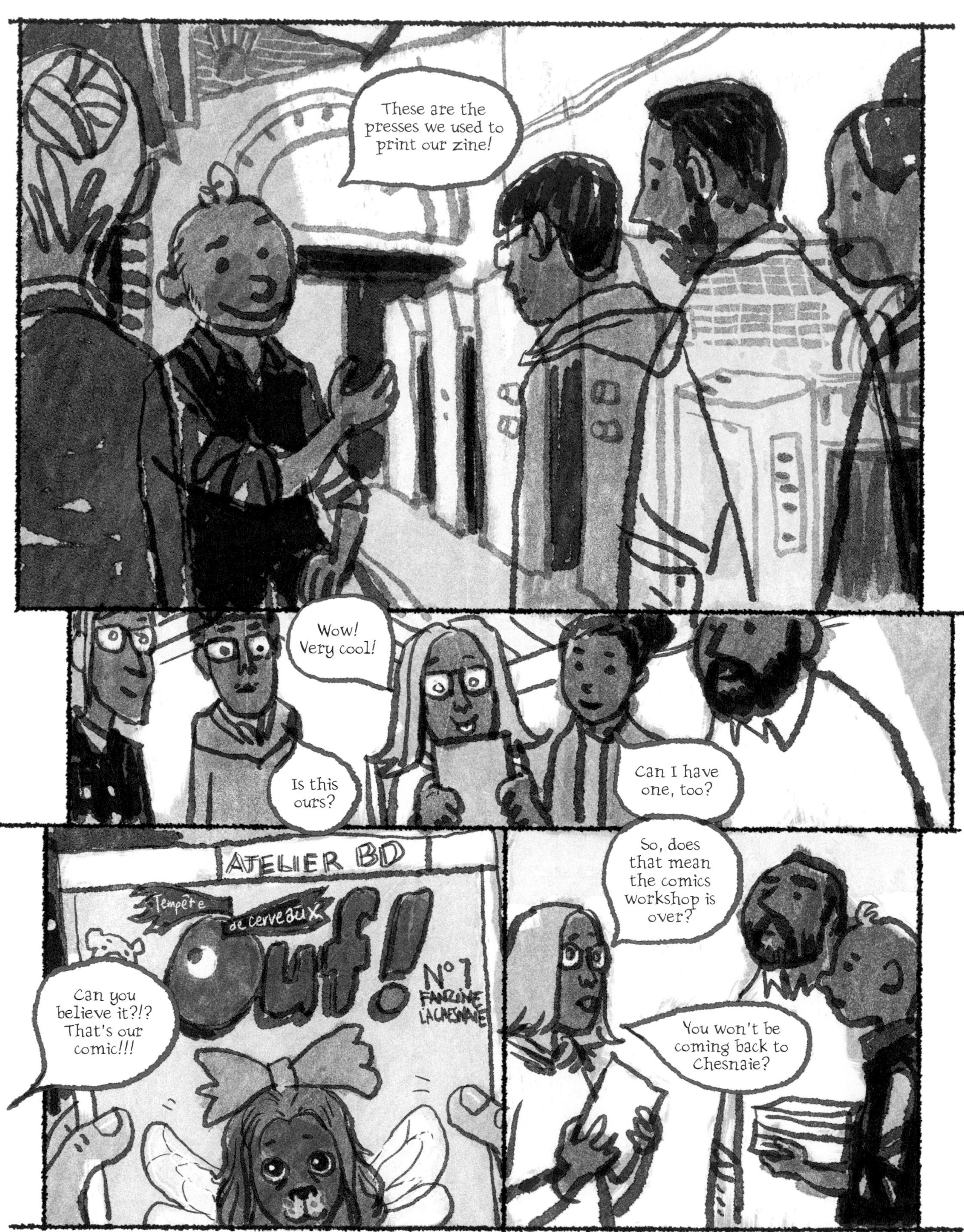
These are the presses we used to print our zine!
Wow! Very cool!
Is this ours?
Can I have one, too?
ATELIER BD
Tempête de cerveaux
Ouf!
N°1 FANZINE LA CHESNAIE
Can you believe it?!? That's our comic!!!
So, does that mean the comics workshop is over?
You won't be coming back to Chesnaie?

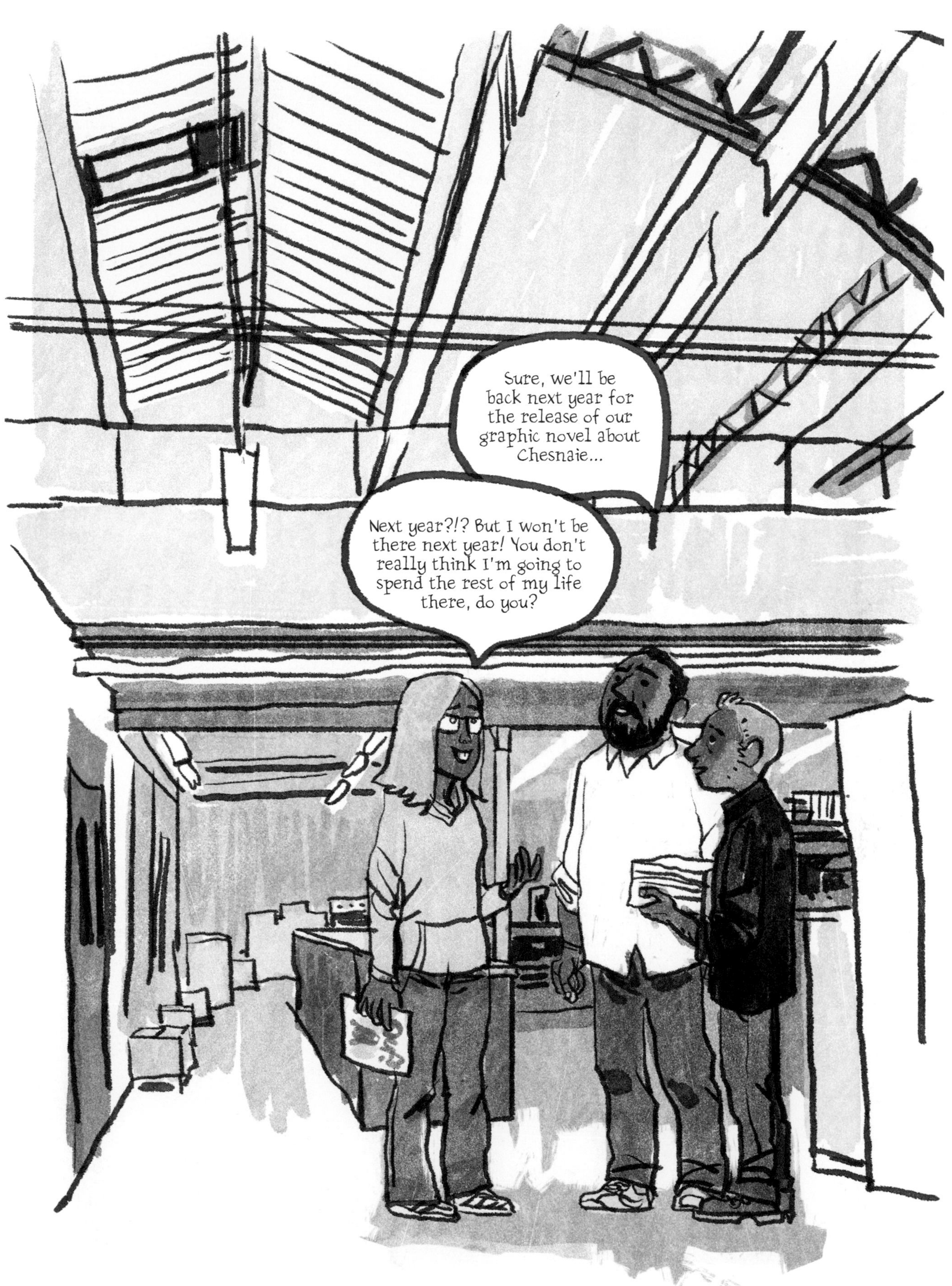
Sure, we'll be back next year for the release of our graphic novel about Chesnaie...
Next year?!? But I won't be there next year! You don't really think I'm going to spend the rest of my life there, do you?

"One must still have chaos within oneself to give birth to a dancing star."
—*Thus Spake Zarathustra*, Friedrich Nietzsche

To Lino and Philémon, two dancing stars.
To Caroline, the chaos in me.

Thanks to Jacqueline (Jean-Yves Duhoo, Marianne Lampel, Etienne Lécroart, Gilles Quétin, and myself) for their willingness to join me in a musical residency at Chesnaie. Is that another story to tell? Dancing stars, in any case!

Greetings to all my friends who supported, encouraged, and advised me. (Stars who...)

Heartfelt gratitude for the evenings we spent at Sonia's and Bruno's. I'll never forget the portrait of Frida Kahlo! (Stars...)

A huge thanks to Gwenaëlle, Aurélien, and the "young Padawan" Virgile, for their hospitality and the good times we had together. Aurélien, star among stars, I love you!

Thank you to the Chesnaie clinic for hosting us, and a special thanks to Sylvie Delagrange, Cathy Charlot, Véronique Beck, and Francois Place. Thanks to Claude Jeangirard for his goodwill.

Thank you to the Chesnaie Club; thank you to the second population; and, of course, thank you to the first!

Thank you to Alain David and Futuropolis. Thank you to the Estienne School for welcoming us and for printing the fanzine *Ouf!*

A huge, huge thanks to Bruno Genini at the Maison de la BD and the entire team at BD Boum for their kindness and expertise.

Jeff Pourquié

Thank you to everyone who warmly welcomed us at the Chesnaie clinic (as well to the others whose refusal made this possible).

Thank you to BD Boum and Bruno Genini (we still owe you five euros).

A special thanks to Cathy for her pep and to Sylvie for her friendship.

A brief and still somewhat annoyed note to the gentleman who asked, with some arrogance and disdain, if "Kierkegaard has a place in comics."

A brotherly hug for Jeff Pourquié, who is as talented as he is kind. I love you, Jeff.

And thanks to Alain David and Futuropolis for their patience, trust, and persistence.

Finally, thanks to Virgile for asking the question at the beginning of this graphic novel.

Aurélien Ducoudray

- Write.
- For whom?
- Write for the dead, for those in the past whom you love.
- Will they read me?
- No!

—Sören Kierkegaard

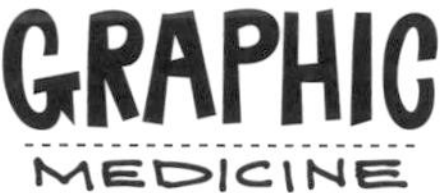

Books in the Graphic Medicine series are inspired by a growing awareness of the value of comics as an important resource for communicating about a range of issues broadly termed "medical." For healthcare practitioners, patients, families, and caregivers dealing with illness and disability, graphic narrative enlightens complicated or difficult experience. For scholars in literary, cultural, and comics studies, the genre articulates a complex and powerful analysis of illness, medicine, and disability and a rethinking of the boundaries of "health." The series includes original comics from artists and non-artists alike, such as self-reflective "graphic pathographies" or comics used in medical training and education, as well as monographic studies and edited collections from scholars, practitioners, and medical educators.

Other titles in the series:

MK Czerwiec, Ian Williams, Susan Merrill Squier, Michael J. Green, Kimberly R. Myers, and Scott T. Smith, *Graphic Medicine Manifesto*

Ian Williams, *The Bad Doctor: The Troubled Life and Times of Dr. Iwan James*

Peter Dunlap-Shohl, *My Degeneration: A Journey Through Parkinson's*

Aneurin Wright, *Things to Do in a Retirement Home Trailer Park: . . . When You're 29 and Unemployed*

Dana Walrath, *Aliceheimers: Alzheimer's Through the Looking Glass*

Lorenzo Servitje and Sherryl Vint, eds., *The Walking Med: Zombies and the Medical Image*

Henny Beaumont, *Hole in the Heart: Bringing Up Beth*

MK Czerwiec, *Taking Turns: Stories from HIV/AIDS Care Unit 371*

Paula Knight, *The Facts of Life*

Gareth Brookes, *A Thousand Coloured Castles*

Jenell Johnson, ed., *Graphic Reproduction: A Comics Anthology*

Olivier Kugler, *Escaping Wars and Waves: Encounters with Syrian Refugees*

Judith Margolis, *Life Support: Invitation to Prayer*

Ian Williams, *The Lady Doctor*

Sarah Lightman, *The Book of Sarah*

Benjamin Dix and Lindsay Pollock, *Vanni: A Family's Struggle through the Sri Lankan Conflict*

Ephameron, *Us Two Together*

Scott T. Smith and José Alaniz, eds., *Uncanny Bodies: Superhero Comics and Disability*

MK Czerwiec, ed., *Menopause: A Comic Treatment*

Susan Merrill Squier and Irmela Marei Krüger-Fürhoff, eds., *PathoGraphics: Narrative, Aesthetics, Contention, Community*

Swann Meralli and Deloupy, *Algériennes: The Forgotten Women of the Algerian Revolution*

Library of Congress Cataloging-in-Publication Data

Names: Ducoudray, Aurélien, 1973– author. | Pourquié, Jeff, illustrator.
Title: The third population / Aurélien Ducoudray and Jeff Pourquié.
Other titles: Troisième population. English | Graphic medicine.
Description: University Park, Pennsylvania : The Pennsylvania State University Press, 2020. | Series: Graphic medicine
Summary: "An exploration, in graphic novel form, of the French psychiatric clinic La Chesnaie. Illustrates the supportive environment where patients and caregivers participate equally in the day-to-day operations of the clinic"—Provided by publisher.
Identifiers: LCCN 2019056974 | ISBN 9780271087177 (cloth)
Subjects: MESH: Hospitals, Psychiatric | Mental Disorders—therapy | Mentally Ill Persons | France | Graphic Novel
Classification: LCC RC439 | NLM WM 17 | DDC 362.2/1—dc23
LC record available at https://lccn.loc.gov/2019056974

Printed in Lithuania
Published by The Pennsylvania State University Press,
University Park, PA 16802-1003
Translated by Kendra Boileau

The Pennsylvania State University Press is a member of the Association of University Presses.

It is the policy of The Pennsylvania State University Press to use acid-free paper. Publications on uncoated stock satisfy the minimum requirements of American National Standard for Information Sciences—Permanence of Paper for Printed Library Material, ANSI Z39.48–1992.